rse the

OXFORD MEDICAL PUBLICATIONS

Emergencies in Sports Medicine

Published and forthcoming titles in the Emergencies in ... series:

Emergencies in Adult Nursing
Edited by Philip Downing

Emergencies in Anaesthesia, Second Edition
Edited by Keith Allman, Andrew McIndoe, and Iain H. Wilson

Emergencies in Cardiology, Second Edition
Edited by Saul G. Myerson, Robin P. Choudhury, and Andrew R.J. Mitchell

Emergencies in Children's and Young People's Nursing
Edited by Edward Alan Glasper, Gillian McEwing, and Jim Richardson

Emergencies in Clinical Medicine
Edited by Piers Page and Greg Skinner

Emergencies in Clinical Radiology
Edited by Richard Graham and Ferdia Gallagher

Emergencies in Clinical Surgery
Edited by Chris Callaghan, J. Andrew Bradley, and Christopher Watson

Emergencies in Critical Care
Edited by Martin Beed, Richard Sherman, and Ravi Mahajan

Emergencies in Mental Health Nursing
Edited by Patrick Callaghan and Helen Waldock

Emergencies in Obstetrics and Gynaecology
Edited by S. Arulkumaran

Emergencies in Oncology
Edited by Martin Scott-Brown, Roy A.J. Spence, and Patrick G. Johnston

Emergencies in Paediatrics and Neonatology
Edited by Stuart Crisp and Jo Rainbow

Emergencies in Palliative and Supportive Care
Edited by David Currow and Katherine Clark

Emergencies in Primary Care
Chantal Simon, Karen O'Reilly, John Buckmaster, and Robin Proctor

Emergencies in Psychiatry
Basant K. Puri and Ian H. Treasaden

Emergencies in Respiratory Medicine
Edited by Robert Parker, Catherine Thomas, and Lesley Bennett

Emergencies in Sports Medicine
Edited by Julian Redhead and Jonathan Gordon

Emergencies in Trauma
Aneel Bhangu, Caroline Lee, and Keith Porter

Head, Neck and Dental Emergencies
Edited by Mike Perry

Medical Emergencies in Dentistry
Nigel Robb and Jason Leitch

Emergencies in Sports Medicine

Edited by

Dr Julian Redhead

FRCP, FCEM, MFSEM

Consultant in Emergency Medicine
Imperial College Healthcare NHS Trust
London, UK

Dr Jonathan Gordon

FRCS, MSc, FCEM, MFSEM

Consultant in Emergency Medicine
Victoria Infirmary
Glasgow, UK

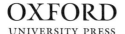

OXFORD
UNIVERSITY PRESS

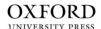

OXFORD

UNIVERSITY PRESS

Great Clarendon Street, Oxford OX2 6DP

Oxford University Press is a department of the University of Oxford.
It furthers the University's objective of excellence in research, scholarship,
and education by publishing worldwide in

Oxford New York

Auckland Cape Town Dar es Salaam Hong Kong Karachi
Kuala Lumpur Madrid Melbourne Mexico City Nairobi
New Delhi Shanghai Taipei Toronto

With offices in

Argentina Austria Brazil Chile Czech Republic France Greece
Guatemala Hungary Italy Japan Poland Portugal Singapore
South Korea Switzerland Thailand Turkey Ukraine Vietnam

Oxford is a registered trade mark of Oxford University Press
in the UK and in certain other countries

Published in the United States
by Oxford University Press Inc., New York

British Library Cataloguing in Publication Data
Data available

Library of Congress Cataloging in Publication Data
Library of Congress Control Number: 2011943540

Typeset by Cenveo, Bangalore, India
Printed in China
on acid-free paper through
Asia Pacific Offset

ISBN 978–0–19–960267–4

10 9 8 7 6 5 4 3 2 1

Preface

Participation in sport and exercise at all levels is recognized as a factor in increasing the medical well being of participants. With the Olympics due in 2012 it is expected that increasing numbers of the population will participate in organized activities.

Healthcare professionals will be expected and encouraged to provide medical care during these events. It is important that these professionals are adequately prepared to provide this care.

A number of excellent courses are available for healthcare professionals to acquire and practice their skills. This text should be viewed as an accompaniment to these courses and to provide immediate access to reliable information at the patients side. The text covers all aspects of the emergencies likely to be encountered and gives important information as to their immediate treatment.

Sport and Exercise Medicine became recognized as a speciality in 2005 with the establishment of a faculty in 2006. Higher specialist training in the speciality began in 2007, with trainees undertaking a 4 year specialist training programme.

The majority of the chapters have been written by trainees within the new speciality, allowing expertise from many different sports to be represented.

We would like to thank them all for their hard work in completing the chapters. We would also like to thank our colleagues within the Emergency Departments for their patience in allowing us to complete the book. The book is dedicated to our wives, Lucy and Julie, and children, Georgina, William, Kate, and Megan.

Acknowledgements

We wish to thank Dr Carl Waldmann for his input and advice for Chapter 9, Head Injuries, and acknowledge Ellen McDougall RGN, Nurse Paralympics GB for the section on autonomic dysreflexia within Chapter 19, Athletes with a disability.

Contents

Contributors

Fiona Burton
ST6 Emergency Medicine
Victoria Infirmary
Glasgow
UK

Eva M. Carneiro
First Team Doctor
Chelsea FC
London
UK

Susan Daisley
Consultant Emergency Medicine
Victoria Infirmary
Glasgow
UK

Sarah Davies
Specialist trainee in Sport and
Exercise Medicine
London Deanery
London
UK

Julie Gordon
Consultant in Emergency Medicine
Crosshouse Hospital
Kilmarnock
UK

Peter L Gregory
The New Dispensary
Warwick
UK

Jonathan Hanson
Consultant in Sport and Exercise
medicine, Scottish Rugby Union.
Department of Emergency
Dr Mackinnon Memorial Hospital
Broadford
Skye
UK

Courtney Kipps
Principal Clinical Teaching Fellow
and Honorary Consultant in Sport
and Exercise Medicine
University College London
London
UK

Pria Krishnasamy
Speciality Registrar in Sport and
Exercise Medicine
London Deanery
London
UK

Jonathan Lacey
Anaesthetic Trainee
Imperial School of Anaesthesia
London
UK

Nina Maryanji
ST 6 Royal Infirmary
Glasgow
UK

Yvonne Moulds
SpR Emergency Medicine
Ayr Hospital
Ayr
UK

Shabaaz Mughal
Club Doctor, Tottenham Hotspur
Football Club
Sport & Exercise Medicine
Consultant Physician
Whipps Cross University Hospital
London
UK

James Noake
Specialist trainee in Sport and
Exercise Medicine
London Deanery
London
UK

Noel Pollock
Consultant in Sport & Exercise
Medicine
UK Athletics London Medical
Officer
Hospital of St John and St Elizabeth
London
UK

John Rogers
Consultant in Sport &
Exercise Medicine
Endurance Medical Officer UKA
UKA National Performance Centre
Loughborough University
Loughborough
UK

Richard Seah
Senior Registrar in Sport &
Exercise Medicine
Royal National Orthopaedic
Hospital NHS Trust
Stanmore
Middlesex
UK

Kevin Thomson
Consultant in Emergency Medicine
Victoria Infirmary
Glasgow
UK

Eleanor Tillett
Honorary Consultant Sport &
Exercise Medicine
University College London
Hospital
London
UK

Symbols and abbreviations

⚠	warning
☙	controversial topic
►►	don't dawdle
►	important
♀	female
♂	male
#	fracture
⌂	website
A&E	Accident & Emergency
ABC	airway, breathing, circulation
ABPI	ankle–brachial pressure index
AC	acromio-clavicular
ACE-I	angiotensin converting enzyme inhibitors
ACL	anterior cruciate ligament
ACS	acute coronary syndrome
AD	autonomic dysflexia
ADH	anti-diuretic hormone
AED	automated external defibrillator
AF	atrial fibrillation
ALS	advanced life support
AMS	acute mountain sickness
AMPLE	allergy, medications, past medical history, last eaten, events preceding
AP	anteroposterior
AS	ankylosing spondylitis
ATLS	advanced trauma life support
AV	atrioventricular
AVPU	Patient alert, Patient responds to verbal stimulus, Patient only responds to painful stimulus, Patient is unresponsive
bd	twice daily
BLS	basic life support
BM	blood glucose monitor
BNF	British National Formulary
BNFC	British National Formulary for Children
BP	blood pressure
CAD	coronary artery disease

CPR	cardiopulmonary resuscitation
CRP	c-reactive protein
CSF	cerebrospinal fluid
CT	computed tomography
CXR	chest X-ray
DIPJ	distal interphalangeal joint
DKA	diabetic keto-acidosis
DMARDs	disease modifying anti-rheumatic drugs
DPL	diagnostic peritoneal lavage
DVT	deep venous thrombosis
EAC	exercise-associated collapse
EAH	exercise-associated hyponatraemia
ECG	electrocardiogram
ECHO	echocardiogram
ED	Emergency Department
EIA	exercise-induced asthma
ERCP	endscopic retrograde cholecystic pancreatogram
ESR	erythrocyte sedimentation rate
ET	Endo-tracheal
FAST	focused assessment with sonography for trauma
FBC	full blood count
FDP	Flexor digitorum profundus
FDS	Flexor digitorum superficialis
FOOSH	fall onto an outstretched hand
GCS	Glasgow Coma Scale
GI	gastrointestinal
GMC	General Medical Council
GTN	glyceryl trinitrate
HACE	high altitude cerebral oedema
HAPE	high altitude pulmonary oedema
HATI	human tetanus immunoglobulin
Hb	haemoglobin
HCM	hypertrophic cardiomyopathy
HIV	human immunodeficiency virus
HOCM	hypertrophic obstructive cardiomyopathy
IBD	Inflammatory bowel disease
IgE	immunoglobin E
IHD	ischaemic heart disease
IM	intramuscular
ITP	idiopathic thrombocytopenic purpura

ITU	intensive therapy unit
IV	intravenous
JVP	jugular venous pressure
LAT	lignocaine, adrenaline, and tetracaine
LIF	left iliac fossa
LMA	laryngeal mask airway
LOC	loss of consciousness
LV	left ventricle
MCL	medial collateral ligament
MD	muscular dystrophy
MDU	Medical Defence Union
MI	myocardial Infarction
MILS	manual in-line immobilization
MRI	magnetic resonance imaging
MS	multiple sclerosis
MTP	metatarso-phalangeal
NAI	non-accidental injury
NCEPOD	National Confidential Enquiry into Patient Outcome and Death
NP	nasopharyngeal
NPA	nasopharyngeal airway
NSAID	non-steroidal anti-inflammatory drug
OGTT	oral glucose tolerance test
OP	oropharyngeal
OPA	oropharyngeal airway
OPT	orthopantomogram
ORIF	open reduction internal fixation
$PaCO_2$	partial pressure of CO_2
PaO_2	partial pressure of O_2
PCL	posterior collateral ligament
PEA	Pulseless electrical activity
PEF	peak expiratory flow
PEFR	peak expiratory flow rate
PIPJ	proximal interphalangeal joint
PMHx	past medical history
po	by mouth
pr	per rectum
PTE	pulmonary embolism
PU	pass urine
RA	rheumatoid arthritis

RBC	red blood cell count
RIF	right iliac fossa
RTA	road traffic accident
RTP	return to play
RUQ	right upper quadrant
SAH	subarachnoid haemorrhage
SARS	severe acute respiratory syndrome
SBP	systolic blood pressure
SC	subcutaneous
SCAT	Sport Concussion Assessment Tool
SCD	sudden cardiac death
SIGN	Scottish Intercollegiate Guidelines Network
SOB	shortness of breath
STI	soft tissue injury
SUFE	slipped upper femoral epiphysis
SVT	supraventrular tachycardias
TB	tuberculosis
VF	ventricular fibrillation
VT	ventricular tachycardia
WADA	world antidoping agency
WBC	white blood cell count
WBGT	wet bulb globe temperature index

Chapter 1

Planning and preparation

Introduction

To fail to prepare is to prepare to fail.

This adage is relevant not only to sporting success, but also when considering planning of medical cover for a sporting event. This chapter outlines the major issues to consider when preparing to cover a sporting event focusing particularly on anticipation and planning for the management of life- and limb-threatening sporting emergencies together with common accident and emergency presentations in a pre-hospital sporting setting.

'There is no place for a token medical presence at sporting events'. This statement issued by the MDU (Medical Defence Union, UK) illustrates the change in attitude over recent years with regard to doctors covering all standards and levels of sporting competition. In previous years, many doctors, physiotherapists, and allied health professionals would volunteer to cover a range of sporting events despite inadequate training, equipment, and personnel. With the development of sport and exercise medicine as a specialty in its own right, the bar is now set considerably higher for doctors and physiotherapists covering these events. The risk of being sued if things go wrong is significant. More importantly, all medical personnel covering sporting events have an ethical responsibility and duty of care to the participants to be properly trained and to make sure they have access to the necessary emergency equipment.

There are many things to take into consideration when agreeing to cover a sporting event and we will cover each one in turn:

Type of sport

Clearly, the type of sport being covered will influence the nature and frequency of injuries seen, and the medical cover, personnel, and equipment required.

In sports, such as motorsport and horse racing, for example, participants are more likely to sustain significant traumatic injuries and there is a requirement to provide personnel and equipment to manage a range of life- and limb-threatening emergencies.

In sports like rugby and football (soccer, American, Gaelic, Australian Rules), again, significant and minor trauma is commonly seen, although athletes also frequently present with over-use type injuries and acute muscle, tendon, and ligamentous injuries.

Sports such as professional boxing and martial arts may see an increased incidence of bleeding and head injuries, whilst diving, rugby, and equestrian see a higher incidence of spinal injuries.

Other sports such as cricket, golf, tennis, swimming, and track and field events, the incidence of life- and limb-threatening emergencies is significantly less. In these non-contact sports, a broad range of over-use type injuries are more commonly seen, but this is not to say that the more significant traumatic/orthopaedic and life-threatening problems do not also occur.

At any sporting event, sudden cardiac events can occur, both in the athletes themselves, but more commonly in excited support staff and spectators. Anaphylaxis may also be encountered in any sport.

⚠ It is important that the doctor or allied health professional covering the event is familiar with the rules of the sport they are covering.

Participants

Clearly, coverage of child, adult, and elderly sporting events will expose the sports medicine practitioner to pathology specific to that age group, and this needs to be accounted for in planning.

When possible, it is extremely useful to have carried out or have access to medical screening data of participants prior to the event. For example, athletes with a previous history of diabetes, epilepsy, cardiac problems, or a history of anaphylactic emergencies should be considered and potential emergencies planned for in advance. Knowledge of the past medical history is particularly important if travelling with a team, and the need for vaccination should also be considered when travelling.

Covering disabled sporting events carries unique challenges and these will be discussed in 📖 Chapter 19.

Responsibilities

When agreeing to cover an event, it is important to make clear from the outset what your responsibilities are. Are you there to cover the athletes only, the spectators/crowd, or both? Are you specifically attached to one team or side? Who is looking after your team's support staff? What other medical personnel will be present? What is their background and experience?

Depending on the size of the event, there will usually be separate first aid or medical cover for spectators. In the UK this is often provided by St John's Ambulance volunteers. At smaller events, where there is no specific doctor to cover spectators you may also be expected to treat people on the sideline. For larger events, it is the responsibility of the doctor covering the sporting event to inform the local A&E department in writing well in advance that the event is taking place. It is useful to reconfirm this closer to the time and to discuss the level of medical cover for the event with one of the senior A&E doctors.

Depending on the nature of the injury, illness, or medical complaint it is sometimes necessary for the doctor covering the athletes to help assess and treat someone from the crowd. One should be wary of being drawn into these situations as it can, in turn, leave the athletes on the field of play uncovered and we would discourage medical personnel specifically covering athletes from getting involved with the crowd unless absolutely necessary, e.g. life-threatening emergency where your help is required.

Venue

It is important to arrive early to look around and get a feel for the venue if you have not worked there before. It is useful to know where various key places and personnel are should you be called to give assistance off the field of play. Key areas to find well in advance of competition are ambulance access, all medical/physio areas, warm-up areas, antidoping rooms, media area, access points to the field of play. Covering events at large stadiums brings its own unique challenges.

The Taylor report was produced by Lord Taylor of Gosforth in the aftermath of the Hillsborough disaster in 1989. In this tragic incident at a football stadium in Sheffield, England, 96 Liverpool FC fans lost their lives. The Taylor report laid out recommendations for safety at sports grounds with specific advice regarding emergency medical cover for the crowd. This was followed by the publication of the Gibson report in 1990. This report stated that, when the number of spectators is expected to be greater than 2000, a doctor trained in advanced first aid is required to be present. The Taylor report recommended that at events where a crowd greater than 5000 is expected, a fully equipped ambulance should be present. It is important to be aware of any major incident plans. We would recommend clarifying what medical cover is in place for the crowd in advance when agreeing to cover athletes/participants at any sporting event.

Environmental conditions

Environmental conditions are an important consideration when planning to cover an event. Of particular concern are the risks of exercising in hot and cold conditions, and of exercising at high altitudes.

Exercising in high temperatures for long periods of time (e.g. marathons, triathlons) increases the risk of conditions such as heat stroke, exercise-associated collapse, and hyponatraemia. Heat stroke and hyponatraemia are medical emergencies, and adequate planning and preparation is crucial in preventing, identifying, and managing these conditions. The wet bulb globe temperature index (WBGT) is used in sport to determine how safe it is to exercise in warm conditions. It takes into account a variety of factors including air temperature, humidity, solar and ground radiation, and wind speed. It is recommended that endurance events should not be held when the WBGT exceeds 28°C. In cooler countries like the UK, the WBGT is not yet widely used at endurance sporting events, even though the above pathologies still occur. Cancelling an event due to adverse environmental conditions can initially bring much criticism both from organizers and participants who have put months into preparation, but ultimately it may be necessary to save lives.

In October 2007, the Chicago marathon was cancelled mid-run due to temperatures soaring to 31°C with one runner dying and hundreds admitted to hospital. In terms of preventative measures, educating participants well in advance on adequate conditioning, acclimatization, cooling, and appropriate rehydration strategies is important. Regular drink and first aid stations are essential. Medical support covering endurance events should be well trained and equipped to deal with emergencies peculiar to hot conditions. Many mass participation endurance events now issue doctors covering the event with rectal thermometers and have point of care analysers at the finish lines to measure serum sodium concentrations. Cold ice baths should be available at the finish for rapid cooling of participants with heat stroke.

Exercising in the cold brings a different set of challenges. Cold pathologies, such as hypothermia and frostbite are more likely to be seen in winter and water-based sports, such as cross-country skiing, mountain climbing, swimming, triathlon, wind surfing, and scuba diving. Endurance events where participants are exposed to milder temperatures for long periods of time with inadequate clothing can also be problematic, e.g. Ironman triathlon.

Hypothermia is defined as a core body temperature of 35°C or lower. As with heat pathologies, it is important that the covering doctor has an adequate thermometer if they are to correctly identify and monitor this condition. We would recommend the use of a low reading rectal thermometer for this purpose. Passive and active rewarming methods should be available when there is a risk of hypothermia, e.g. dry blankets, space blankets, hot drinks, hot air blankets, and the application of heat packs to the torso, axillae, and groin. Again, education of participants well in advance on preventative strategies and written guidance for well-trained medical staff is an essential part of planning.

We will discuss the management of environmental emergencies in more detail in 📖 Chapter 5.

Medical personnel required

Demand on medical services from previous similar event coverage will help guide the organizing medical officer when planning the number of doctors, physiotherapists, paramedics and ambulance technicians, nurses, first aiders, and sports massage therapists required.

It is important to take into account the expected number of participants and available epidemiological literature when planning medical cover. At larger national and international sporting events, teams often have their own doctors and physiotherapists who work alongside medical staff responsible for the event.

A co-ordinated multidisciplinary team approach is an important part of event coverage. It is useful to meet the different members of the team before the event starts to make introductions and raise any concerns.

We would strongly recommend practicing emergency scenarios with the different members of the team before the event starts, e.g. spinal injury, fracture dislocation of ankle, anaphylaxis, cardiac arrest, etc. This serves several purposes—it refreshes emergency care skills, it helps clarify people's roles, it familiarizes staff with the medical equipment they may need to use, and it helps people who may have never met before interact and get to know each other.

Transportation

Imagine trying to carry a 16-stone rugby player with a badly sprained ankle 200 m to the warmth of the nearest dressing room and one soon understands the importance of assistance with transport. Simple items such as a stretcher or a set of crutches to transfer a casualty from the field of play should be readily available.

For time-critical emergencies, an ambulance should be sought to transport the athlete/patient to the most appropriate medical facility or hospital. Larger sporting events will usually have a fully equipped ambulance and paramedics in attendance at the venue. It may seem like common sense, but the covering medical personnel should know the emergency service number relevant to the country they are working in (i.e. 999 in UK). One should be ready to provide an accurate address and be able to give relevant information about the casualty to the ambulance control centre. If one is working in an area where it is likely to take a significant length of time to transport a casualty to hospital then they should be proficient in providing advanced life support in a pre-hospital setting.

To save valuable time, it is often useful to have someone at the entrance to the sporting venue to meet and direct the ambulance to the casualty.

Communication

As with working in any medical specialty, the practice of good communication skills can make the difference between a happy, competent, and well co-ordinated team of professionals and a disorganized, inefficient, and ineffective shambles! When covering certain sports, e.g. horse racing, motorsport, medical staff may be large distances apart and effective communication devices are crucial.

A charged mobile phone with good network signal coverage is one of the most useful items to have in your possession when covering a sporting event. It is useful to exchange mobile numbers with other medical personnel and key officials covering the event. Many larger events will also have walkie-talkies (hand-held radio transceivers) for medical staff and officials. In noisy venues with large crowds it is useful to have an earpiece connection or even headphones. It is important to test these devices before usage to make sure one is using the correct channel and that the volume is adequate.

Equipment and medication

Items will vary depending on the practitioner's own preference, the type of sport covered, local supplies, number of participants, and duration of event coverage. Pitch side doctors and physiotherapists will often carry a small grab bag (Fig. 1.1) with commonly used emergency equipment and medication. It is important to be mindful of the world antidoping agency (WADA) code and its banned substance list when preparing medication supplies for a sporting event. The following list is neither prescriptive nor exhaustive.

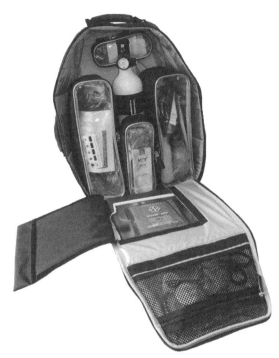

Fig. 1.1 Pitch side resuscitation bag—'Sportpromote'.

- Effective means of communication with paramedics—own mobiles and walkie talkies
- Designated first aid or treatment room with the ability to provide privacy for the casualty
- Automated external defibrillator (AED)—defibrillator
- Emergency equipment including oro- and nasopharyngeal airways, laryngeal mask apparatus, O_2, Entonox®, bag valve mask, range of cervical collars, spinal board, selection of intravenous (IV) cannulae, fracture splints
- IV fluids (normal saline 1 L) IV giving sets, selection of cannulae, and venflon skin fixers
- Resus pocket masks
- EpiPen® or generic alternative (or adrenaline 1:1000 solution 1 mg in 1 mL—1 ampoule)
- Otoscope/ophthalmoscope
- Stethoscope
- Sphygmomanometer

- Mirror
- Thermometer
- Blood glucose testing meter
- British National Formulary (BNF)/BNF for Children (BNFC)
- Bottles of water for rehydration and cleaning
- Peak flow meter
- Salbutamol inhalers
- Compatible spacer device
- Beclometasone inhaler
- Portable nebulizer
- Salbutamol nebules
- Ipratropium bromide nebulizer solution
- Prednisolone tablets
- Beclometasone spray
- Paracetamol
- Codeine
- Ibuprofen
- Diclofenac
- Voltarol Emulgel®
- Loperamide
- Metoclopramide po
- Metoclopramide—10 mg 2-mL amp for injection
- Gaviscon® liquid
- Omeprazole
- Broad spectrum antibiotics
- Benzylpenicillin 600 mg for intramuscular (IM) injection—Crystapen® 2 vial GP pack
- Hydrocortisone 1% cream
- Strepsils® or other throat lozenges
- Disposable tongue depressors
- Urinalysis Multistix®
- Fluorescein eye drops 1%
- Tetracaine eye drops 1%
- Ear drops—Otomize®
- Bandages, slings/triangular bandage, sterile gauze pads, cling film, providone-iodine, dressing packs, dressings—dry, moist, and non-stick
- Scalpels
- Needles—greens, blues and orange
- 2, 5, and 10-mL syringes
- Suture kits
- 3/0, 4/0 and 5/0 sutures
- Steri-strips®
- Staple suture pack
- Anti-tetanus prophylaxis
- Nasal plugs
- Sterets
- Lidocaine 1%
- Bupivicaine 0.5%
- Range of Tubigrip® sizes
- Variety of tapes
- Collar and cuff

- Chlorphenamine for injection 10 mg/mL
- Cetirizine or other antihistamine
- Hydrocortisone for injection—Efcortesol® 5-mL ampoule
- Diazemuls® 5 mg/mL—2 mL ampoule
- Diazepam rectal tube 2.5 mL (10 mg) tube
- Saline or water for injection—10 mL
- GlucoGel® gel
- Glucagon for injection 1 mg
- Glucose for IV injection 20%, 50 mL
- Bib clearly identifying role
- Identification with assured access to all areas
- Bag for kit
- Vinyl or latex examination gloves
- Injury reporting sheets with carbon copy paper
- Sharps disposal bins
- Clinical waste bags
- Heavy gauge scissors
- Emergency cricothyroidotomy kit
- Morphine sulphate for intravenous injection—10 mg/mL × 10 (this will need to written on a separate script and kept in a locked case). It requires secure storage outside of competition times and if carried should be obtained using form FP10CDF
- Naloxone 2 mL (800 mcg) prefilled syringe
- Glyceryl trinitrate (GTN) spray 400 mcg/dose
- Aspirin 300 mg
- Adrenaline 1 in 10,000—1 mg in 10 mL for injection
- Hyoscine butylbromide
- Ice bags
- Dental kit
- Sport concussion assessment tool (SCAT) card

You will need to ensure you are familiar with all the equipment you take with you or are provided with at the event, i.e. AED. Remember that controlled drugs, whilst useful, are also potentially problematic (i.e. keeping secure, passing through airport security) and you should give serious consideration to such issues when travelling abroad.

In terms of getting your own kit together it is perhaps easier to think about what you require to manage your patient with respect to the airway, breathing, circulation (A, B, C), and break down the other items into either the medical or surgical items you will need. Keeping these different items in 3 separate smaller bags within 1 large bag will help to ensure you have everything to hand when you need it.

Do not be too concerned about bringing complex items of kit at the expense of remembering the simple things, i.e. gloves, sharps bins, etc.

Documentation

Documentation in a sporting context may be difficult, with many consultations taking place in a public place where writing detailed notes and recording medical information electronically may simply not be possible. The use of hand-held electronic devices that link to computers can be useful for the more IT literate practitioner. It is often necessary to document consultations many minutes or even hours after the assessment took place, and some form of *aide memoire*, such as a notepad, is often helpful. Most professional sports clubs now use encrypted online electronic medical records, which can be accessed and added to from anywhere in the world with Internet access.

In the medico-legal age we now work in, good documentation is increasingly important. In emergencies, good documentation is particularly important for communicating with medical staff taking over care in a hospital setting. Injury reporting sheets, as used by paramedics, with sections for primary and secondary surveys together with carbon copy paper are useful for this purpose.

Headed note paper and a prescription pad are also useful.

Security/identification

At major championships, participants, officials, and medical staff are issued with accreditation passes. These will usually have numbers to signify which areas can be accessed. It is important to check that you will be able to access any area where your assistance may be needed. This usually means access all areas, although this is not always possible. In life-threatening emergencies (particularly in foreign countries where language barriers can be a problem) one may need to get access to a competitor quickly to ensure proper medical care is established. It is useful to plan for these eventualities in advance and anything that easily identifies you as medical personnel is usually all that is needed. In the current political climate, large sporting events can be a target for terrorists and it is useful to be familiar with any major incident plans.

Indemnity

Medical staff covering sporting events should discuss their indemnity cover with their defence organization in advance to make sure they are covered for any potential legal action. National governing bodies in sport may also be able to offer advice in this difficult area. In professional sport, indemnity insurance can prove costly, but should never be ignored.

Further reading

Allen M (2000). Medical officers at sporting events. *Journal of the Medical Defence Union*, **16**:8–9.

Gibson RM (1990). *Report of the Medical Working Party*. HMSO, London.

Lord Justice Taylor (1990). *Final Report into the Hillsborough Stadium Disaster*. HMSO, London.

🏃 www.sportpromote.co.uk/medical-bag.

General approach to the injured or unwell athlete

Introduction

Proper planning prevents poor performance.

Doctors and other healthcare professionals will be called upon to deal with both traumatic and medical emergencies. The general principles in the treatment of these patients are the same. Often there will be little or no information available to the attending professional, and so the priorities must be to restore the patient's vital functions first, and then, when time allows a more detailed head to toe assessment can be carried out.

The assessment, by definition, must be rapid and accompanied by action. It must also be thorough and miss nothing out. The prioritized assessment, which was first comprehensively described in the advanced trauma life support course, lends itself to the treatment of the critically ill patient, but should also be used in the initial assessment of all patients. This chapter will give an overview of the assessment but details will also be available in subsequent chapters.

Preparation
- Ensure you have equipment available to you to deal with the emergencies you might encounter
- Ensure that you are familiar with any equipment provided at an event
- Ensure you are familiar with evacuation routes for casualties
- Ensure you are aware of local facilities to continue the treatment of your patients and how to access them in an emergency
- Ensure that you regularly practice scenarios for the conditions you are likely to encounter, ideally with the other healthcare resources you will usually have available
- Ensure all personnel involved in treating a patient are aware of the principles of initial assessment and management, as well as the potential resources involved in the care of these patients
- Ensure that you understand when it is safe or appropriate to approach a patient while on the field of play. It is often best to discuss this with any official, ensuring that emergency care can be delivered in a safe environment and in a timely manner.

Rapid assessment and synchronous resuscitation
Obtain a brief history from the patient, relatives, or witnesses. This can be done while beginning to assess the patient. The mnemonic AMPLE is useful in this regard.
- **A**—allergies
- **M**—medication
- **P**—past medical history
- **L**—last meal
- **E**—events leading up to the need for medical help.

Check whether the patient is conscious
Always approach a patient involved in trauma as if they may have a cervical spine injury. Before talking to the patient hands should be placed around the head to provide in line immobilization of the neck. This is best provided by approaching a prone patient from their head end. Approaching from the side

and calling to a patient is likely to provoke the reaction of turning the head, which may exacerbate a spinal injury.

- If the patient is conscious then introduce yourself and reassure the patient. Patients who survive critical situations will often remember calm words directed to them for a long time afterwards
- If the patient is unconscious call for help and continue the assessment
- Ensure that you have allocated a single person to call an ambulance, asking them to confirm to you when this has been achieved
- Initially check to see if the patient is breathing. If they are not breathing then proceed directly to treat them for cardiac arrest—detailed in 📖 Chapter 3.

A: assess the airway

- If the patient is able to speak normally, then the airway is patent. Ensure that the voice is not 'hoarse', or that stridor is present from upper airway obstruction, or injury
- If stridor or hoarseness is present, then urgent transfer to an emergency department (ED) is indicated. The patient should be kept calm and given high flow oxygen. Do not attempt to examine the throat. No surgical airway is indicated in a conscious patient
- If the patient is unconscious then the airway can be opened by a jaw thrust manoeuvre:
  - Direct visualization of the oral cavity can be made and suction, if available, used to clear any secretions/blood, etc.
  - Keep the tip of the suction catheter under direct vision at all times
  - Large objects can be removed from the mouth, such as mouth guards, but no blind finger sweeps should be undertaken
  - Ensure enough personnel are available to log roll the patient in the event of vomiting–ensure they understand their individual role in the event of requiring a log roll.

B: assess the breathing

- Count the respiratory rate and assess the effort required in breathing, such as pain, extramuscular use (in-drawing, recession, tracheal tug, etc.)
- Examine the chest for abnormal movement patterns such as asymmetrical chest movement or evidence of a flail segment
- Check for tenderness
- If possible listen to the chest for additional sounds such as wheeze or absence of sounds suggestive of a pneumothorax. If a pneumothorax is suspected check for evidence of tension by ensuring the trachea is central suggesting no abnormal mediastinal shift
- For treatment of chest injuries see 📖 Chapter 3; however, the majority of chest injuries are treated initially with high flow oxygen only
- If a tension pneumothorax is suspected then it can be relieved by a needle decompression, if the practitioner has been trained in the procedure.

In the athletic population it is appropriate to treat all patients with a potential chest injury with high flow oxygen.

C: assess the circulation

- Feel the pulse and count the rate
- If the radial pulse is palpable then it may be assumed that the systolic Blood Pressure (BP) is over 90 mmHg. If a pulse is not palpable then intravenous fluids (IV) may be beneficial and simple manoeuvres such as raising the legs would be appropriate, depending on the injuries to the pelvis, or lower limbs
- Examine for distended neck veins. If they are distended then consider a diagnosis of tension pneumothorax if other signs are present:
  - Evidence of chest injury
  - Respiratory distress
  - Reduced breath sounds
  - Hyper-resonance to the chest on the affected side.

Shock can be divided into 5 mechanisms
- Hypovolaemic
- Neurogenic (due to spinal injury and characterized by decreased blood pressure, but a normal or slow heart rate)
- Obstructive (e.g. tension pneumothorax)
- Cardiogenic
- Septic.

In sports medicine the first three are the most likely. It must be remembered that athletes have a large cardiac reserve and will often have a bradycardic resting pulse. In these circumstances a 'normal' heart rate may be indicative of early 'shock'.

The treatment of shock includes applying pressure to external bleeding points, IV fluids if the radial pulse is absent, raising the legs if appropriate, giving high flow oxygen via a non re-breath mask (one with a reservoir bag).

D: assess neurological disability

This is best assessed using the AVPU scale:
- **A**—patient alert
- **V**—patient responds to verbal stimulus
- **P**—patient only responds to painful stimulus
- **U**—patient is unresponsive.

If the patient is alert but has suffered a head injury then further analysis for concussion should be carried out using an appropriate scoring system (see 📖 p.116).

Always assume a neck injury, and protect the cervical spine unless you have clinically examined, and cleared any possible injury.

E: expose the patient

Always ensure that all potential injuries have been excluded. This is best done by a rapid head to toe examination as indicated by the injury pattern. Ensure the patient remains warm.

Continuing evaluation of the patient

- If the patient's condition deteriorates always reassess the patients ABCDE, and treat appropriately
- Arrange for evacuation of the patient to an appropriate medical area while awaiting further assistance from the ambulance service or other appropriate medical care
- Evacuation of the patient should be carried out assuming a spinal injury whenever appropriate. The log roll of the patient is an essential element of this process and whenever possible the team likely to be involved in this manoeuvre should practice together prior to the event.

The log roll

This is an important manoeuvre in the care of any patient with a suspected spinal injury, including an unconscious patient. This involves 4 personnel to carry out the roll and at least one person to examine the patient or manoeuvre extraction equipment into place.

Person 1

This person provides in line immobilization of the cervical spine. They are also in charge of the whole manoeuvre and therefore have additional responsibilities.

- Ensure safety of the patient at all times
- Ensure all personnel are briefed as to the mechanism of the roll
- Ensure all staff have correct hand positions
- Ensure all staff are briefed as to the correct instructions for the roll. This is often best expressed by 'ready, brace, roll'—where the manoeuvre starts on the instruction roll
- Ensure the patient is briefed.

Person 2

Ensure the arms are placed across the chest, and then position hands so that one is placed on the opposite shoulder to where this person is placed, and the other on the pelvis.

Person 3

One hand is placed on the pelvis next to person 2 hand (sometimes they cross hands for stability). The other is placed under the patients opposite thigh.

Person 4

One hand is placed under the thigh next to person 3 hand. The other hand is placed under the opposite calf. All hands should be placed on bony areas for stability.

Extremity trauma

This will also be covered in subsequent chapters, but the principles of treatment are:

- Check for a pulse
- If obvious deformity and a pulse is palpable then do not attempt reduction unless trained to do so
- If obvious deformity and no pulse, then if the practitioner feels comfortable in gently reducing the area to an anatomical position, this can be attempted. If a pulse is regained then splint the limb in that position. If no pulse is achieved then ensure that medical personnel summoned are aware of the absence of a pulse
- Splint the limb—this is usually achieved through the use of a box splint, although vacuum splints may also be used. It is important to practice with the equipment available prior to an event
- If the wound is open, i.e. a breach of the skin has occurred, then a clean dressing should be placed over the area. If possible a photograph should be taken, so that other attending practitioners can review the wound without removing the dressing
- Analgesia should be provided. This is often best given by the use of Entonox®, or opiates if monitoring is available.

Entonox®

This is a 50:50 mixture of NO and O_2. It is delivered through a patient demand valve. It provides analgesia, but does not render the patient unconscious. It has a short half-life, so constant inhalation while in pain will be necessary.

Contraindications to use:

- Head injury
- Chest injury
- Suspected injury due to diving to depths.

Relative contraindications to use

- Patients where air may be trapped in an organ, e.g. post some ophthalmological operations, sinusitis, etc.
- In a cold environment it is necessary to mix the gases, which will separate under 4°C. This involves inversion of the bottle at least three times.

Opiates

- Fentanyl 'lollipops' are increasingly being used in the pre-hospital environment
- They provide excellent analgesia without the need for IV access
- Patients must have appropriate monitoring available and be trained in their use
- Storage of the drug must comply with regulations regarding the storage of controlled drugs.

Cardiorespiratory arrest

Basic life support: an introduction

The most recent European Resuscitation Council Guidelines were published in October 2010. The key message from these guidelines remains the provision of effective CPR and early defibrillation where available.

These guidelines do not fundamentally change from the greater emphasis on chest compressions that was the basis of the 2005 guidelines. The aim is making these as uninterrupted as possible. The ratio of compressions to ventilations therefore remains 30:2.

- Once CPR has started it should not stop unless the victim shows signs of life, such as return of consciousness, in addition to a return of normal breathing
- Within a sports setting, there is also the potential of concurrent trauma and so manual in-line immobilization (MILS) should be carried out to protect the cervical spine during resuscitation attempts if injury is suspected:
  - This will not be possible with only 1 provider of life support
  - If MILS is interfering with quality of resuscitation, and the risk of neck injury is considered to be low then it may be discarded
- On field cardiac arrest classically occurs as an 'off the ball' syncopal collapse
- Recent high profile cases such as Marc Vivian Foe, Miklos Feher, and Antonia Puerta continue to highlight the issue of sudden cardiac death:
  - They demonstrate the need to ensure adequate training of pitchside medical staff in life-support, as well as access to appropriate medical kit including defibrillators
  - The case of the collapse of Evander Sno who was successfully defibrillated at the pitchside also shows the invaluable benefit to be gained by being trained in life support and having the appropriate kit.

Remember that basic life support (BLS) is only basic in terms of the levels of kit required to perform it. It is a vital part of the cardiac arrest management and you should be familiar with the algorithms so that you are comfortable in performing it.

☠️ Adult basic life support

This is based upon the European Resuscitation Guidelines 2010. Follows an ABC approach (Fig. 3.1):
- Check safe to approach
- Speak to casualty 'Are you alright?'
- Stimulate the casualty for responsiveness through gentle shaking, but if a potential spinal injury is suspected consider a very gentle stimulus above and below the clavicle.

Outcome 1: patient responds
Leave him where he is unless he is in danger. Try to find out what's wrong. Reassess regularly.

Outcome 2: no response
- Shout for help and turn patient onto their back. Pay some consideration to the chance of a potential spinal injury when moving the athlete, but not if it interferes with ongoing management
- If still no response:
  - Call for help
  - Ensure an ambulance has been called and an AED requested
  - Ensure you have access to your resuscitation equipment.
- **A** Open the airway via head tilt, chin lift, or jaw thrust
- **B** Place your cheek above the casualty's mouth:
  - Look (at the chest)
  - Listen (for breathing)
  - Feel (breath on your cheek) for normal breathing for *no more* than 10 s. If you have any doubt then act as if *not* normal
- **C** Those who are skilled at palpating the carotid pulse can do so whilst assessing breathing. Otherwise look for signs of circulation, such as the athletes colour and normal breathing.

Outcome 1: patient breathing normally
- Place patient to the recovery position
- Await ambulance
- Reassess breathing regularly.

Outcome 2: not breathing normally
- Ensure an ambulance has been called/requested, leave the patient as a last measure to contact help
- If the casualty is not breathing normally, assume there is no circulation and commence cardiac compressions at a ratio of 30 compressions to 2 rescue breaths and at a rate of compression of 100–120/min
- Continue until:
  - The patient shows signs of a regaining consciousness *and* starts to breathe normally
  - Until more skilled help arrives
  - Until you are exhausted.

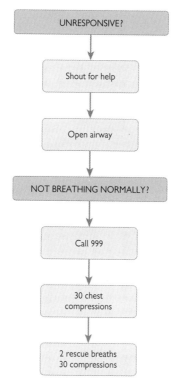

Fig. 3.1 Adult basic life support algorithm. Reproduced with the kind permission of the Resuscitation Council (UK).

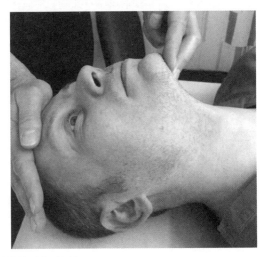

Fig. 3.2 Head tilt, chin lift.

Head tilt, chin lift

- Unsuitable in suspected c-spine injury.
- Place one hand across the forehead and two fingers of the other under the point of the chin.
- Lift up under the chin and support the forehead – 'Sniffing the morning air' position—see Fig. 3.2.

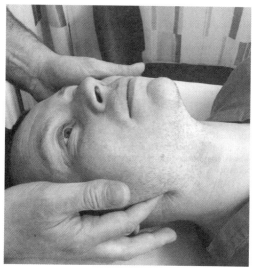

Fig. 3.3 Jaw thrust.

Jaw thrust

- Not recommended for lay individuals
- Place both thumbs on the zygomas with the fingers behind the angles of the mandible
- Lift the mandible forward thus elevating the tongue away from the soft palate—see Fig. 3.3.

Cardiac compressions

- Ratio of 30 compressions: 2 breaths
- Kneel by the side of the victim
- Place the heel of one hand in the centre of the chest with the other hand upon it
- Press firmly down 5–6 cm. Allow full recoil of chest after compression
- Return hands to starting position without losing contact with the chest
- Repeat 30 times
- Perform compressions at a rate of 100–120/min.

Rescue breaths
- Pinch nose with the index finger and thumb of the hand resting on the patient's forehead
- Allow mouth to open, but maintain chin lift
- Form a seal around victim's lips with your mouth
- Blow steadily into mouth
- Watch chest rise for 1 s. (This is shorter than in previous guidelines)
- Repeat and return hands to chest compression position, thereby minimizing interruptions. The 2 breaths should take no more than 5 s.

What if the chest doesn't rise on rescue breaths?
- Check mouth for obstruction
- Is there adequate neck extension?
- Do not attempt more than two breaths before returning to compressions.

Tired
- Evidence suggests the quality of compressions falls in tired rescuers, so swap after 2 min
- *Compression only:* perform cardiopulmonary resuscitation (CPR) at a rate of 100–120/min
- Entirely reasonable for those unwilling to do mouth to mouth ventilation.

Risk to rescuer from mouth to mouth resuscitation
- Very small
- Occasional report of tuberculosis or severe acute respiratory syndrome (SARS)
- No HIV transmission reported
- Consider use of a pocket mask with valve.

Upon arrival of a defibrillator
- Connect pads to patient and shock *immediately* if advised.
- **Note:** 2° min of CPR are no longer performed before defibrillating in the case of an unwitnessed arrest out of hospital.

Drowning
Five initial rescue breaths followed by 1 min of chest compressions is recommended *before* going to get help.

☺: Paediatric basic life support

The main difference between the cardiac arrest suffered by a child compared with an adult is that the aetiology is usually primarily cardiac in adults whereas in children it is more commonly respiratory resulting in a secondary cardiac arrest (see Fig. 3.4).

Initial assessment is along the same A, B, C guidelines as for the adult.

- Check safe to approach
- Speak to casualty 'Are you alright?'
- Stimulate the casualty for responsiveness through gentle shaking, but if a potential spinal injury is suspected consider a very gentle stimulus above and below the clavicle.

Outcome 1: patient responds
- Leave him where he is unless he is in danger
- Try to find out what's wrong
- Reassess regularly.

Outcome 2: no response
- Shout for help and turn patient onto their back. Pay some consideration to the chance of a potential spinal injury when moving the athlete, but not if it interferes with ongoing management.
- If still no response:
  - Call for help
  - Ensure an ambulance has been called
  - Ensure you have access to your resuscitation equipment
- Upon confirming arrest give 5 initial rescue breaths before starting compressions
- If you are on your own, perform 1 min of CPR *before* going for help
- Ratio of 15 compressions: 2 breaths
- Compress the chest by *at least* one-third of its depth. This is a subtle difference to highlight and reassure that it is safe to compress a child's chest.
  - Use two fingers for an infant under 1 year
  - Use one or two hands for a child over 1 year as needed to achieve depth of compression. Rate is at least 100, but not greater than 120/min
- If you are struggling to achieve ventilations then consider foreign body or repositioning of the child's head or neck to a more 'neutral' position compared to the 'sniffing the morning air' position used in adults
- A standard defibrillator can be safely used for children over 8 years of age:
  - Between the ages of 1 and 8 years paediatric pads or mode if available on the AED should be used if possible. If not available then use the AED as it comes.
  - For an infant under 1-year-old, if no other manually adjustable defibrillator is available then an AED should still be used if the rhythm is shockable.

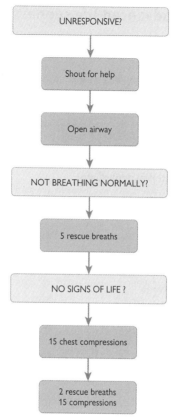

Fig. 3.4 Paediatric basic life support. Reproduced with the kind permission of the Resuscitation Council (UK).

☢: **Adult advanced life support**

- Initially follows the BLS algorithm, but rather than continuing to exhaustion, there is reassessment at 2 min intervals. The difference is to intervene with early defibrillation and possibly drug therapy if appropriate
- The crux of advanced life support (ALS) is deciding if the rhythm is shockable (ventricular fibrillation, ventricular tachycardia) or non-shockable (asystole or pulseless electrical activity) whereupon a separate limb of the algorithm develops for each (Fig. 3.5)
- 2 min of 30 compressions to 2 ventilations roughly equates to 10 breaths, i.e. 5 cycles of 30:2
- CPR should continue even while the defibrillator is charging, thus minimizing the loss of compressions pre-shock.

Automated external defibrillator

- This device is capable of analysing the underlying cardiac rhythm and advising the user whether to deliver a shock to attempt to re-store normal circulation
- They come in a variety of complexities, but are very reliable and a safe way of partially skilled users performing defibrillation. Training is *not* required in order to use these
- AED should be requested at the same time that the ambulance is called.

Abnormal rhythms

Ventricular fibrillation (VF)

- Random uncoordinated myocyte activity
- Always fatal unless defibrillated.

Ventricular tachycardia (VT)

- The beat is being led by ventricular muscle rather than the natural pacemaker of the heart—the sinoatrial node
- A rhythm of varying degrees of organization, so it may or may not provide a blood pressure
- An inefficient rhythm that will eventually decay to VF.

Asystole

- No electrical activity in the heart
- Cannot be defibrillated
- Has a very poor outcome.

Pulseless electrical activity (PEA)

- Normal electrical activity of the heart is uncoupled from its mechanical action
- Usually a complex cause that needs to be addressed
- A non-shockable rhythm.

Drugs

Delivery should be intravenous (IV). If IV access is unavailable then the intraosseous route is recommended. The tracheal route is no longer recommended.

Adrenaline 1 mg

- 1 in 10,000 IV. 10 mL = 1 mg
- Given in the shockable side of the ALS algorithm immediately after the third shock and every 3–5 min thereafter
- Works as a powerful peripheral vasoconstrictor, thus promoting blood flow to vital organs
- In the non-shockable side of the algorithm it is given immediately, then every 3–5 min.

Amiodarone 300 mg

Given at the same time as adrenaline after the 3rd shock.

Atropine 3 mg IV

No longer routinely recommended in asystole or PEA.

Prolonged or non-shockable arrests

Consider the '4H's and 4T's and address these issues as necessary.

- *Hypothermia:* caused by immersion or exposure
- *Hyper/hypokalaemia:* think medication (diuretics)
- *Hypoxia:* common in general population and children
- *Hypovolaemia:* recent trauma or occult bleeding?
- *Thromboembolic disease:* recent flight?
- *Toxins:* recreational drugs?
- *Tamponade:* recent chest trauma?
- *Tension pneumothorax:* recent trauma or chest pain?

Advanced airway management

- Most airways will be managed with effective basic manoeuvres and a bag valve mask
- Equipment such as a nasopharyngeal airway (NPA) or an oropharygeal airway (OPA) are useful tools
- In ALS, endotracheal intubation is the 'gold standard' method of addressing hypoxia
- However, intubation is a complex skill that needs to be performed frequently to ensure safe insertion; it is thus out of the scope for many sports medicine practitioners
- An intermediate stage of airway management involves the laryngeal mask airway (LMA)—effectively a 'hands-free' face mask that is inserted to sit on top of the glottis
- LMAs need little skill or practice to use and are a useful tool in the sports setting. A more modern variant is the i-gel thermogel device.

Key advanced life support points/ changes

- Minimize interruptions to chest compressions. Rhythmic compression maintains coronary perfusion pressure during diastole. This pressure falls rapidly when compressions cease. Continue chest compressions whilst waiting for the defibrillator to charge. Each minutes delay in defibrillation results in a 10% decreased chance that resuscitation will be successful
- Compress the chest 5–6cm at a rate of 100–120 per min
- Rescue breaths take 1 s to inflate the chest
- Atropine is no longer recommended.

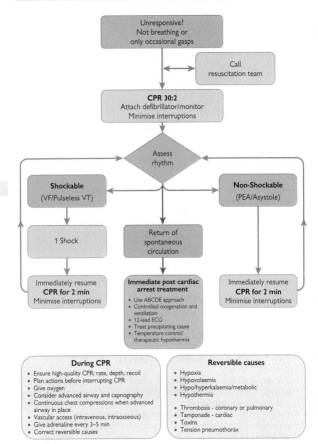

Fig. 3.5 Adult advanced life support algorithm. Reproduced with the kind permission of the Resuscitation Council (UK).

Planning for critical care incidents at sporting events

- There are now many courses in the UK that provide sports pre-hospital critical care skills. (E.g. Remo/Area/Immofp/Phtcc/ Scrumcaps/Sportpromote)
- All these courses advise that availability of critical care kit and appropriate training to use it should be an essential part of match day planning
- Remember that the guidelines suggest attempted defibrillation should occur within 3 min of a cardiac arrest, therefore having a defibrillator locked in someone's car is insufficient!
- Critical care kit needs to be in the immediate vicinity of where athletic activity is taking place and skill updates need to be frequently repeated by all members of the wider medical team.

Further reading

Resuscitation Council.

🔗 www.resus.org.uk.

Athletes with pre-existing conditions

⚙ Diabetes mellitus

▶▶ For the management of hypoglycaemia and diabetic keto-acidosis (DKA) see 📖 p.92.

- Diabetes is a chronic condition characterized by a lack of endogenous insulin. This results in chaotic blood glucose levels
- Diabetes occurs in approximately 4% of the UK population. There has been a notable increase in diagnosed cases in the last 10 years, although this varies widely depending on different population groups
- Approximately 10–15% of diabetics are insulin dependent with 85–90% either dietary or tablet controlled
- Exercise is important in the diabetic population due to the secondary effects diabetes has on end organ disease and its association with such conditions as ischaemic heart disease, hypertension, and peripheral vascular disease
- As a team clinician you may be called to treat someone who is suffering the effects of diabetes who is either known to be diabetic, or presenting for the first time
- A history of lethargy, polyuria, and polydispsia are classically described symptoms for someone presenting with diabetes. More subtle presentations such as recurring skin infections should also raise the possibility of the diagnosis
  - Always test blood sugar in an athlete in whom you suspect diabetes may be a possibility or the cause of the symptoms presenting to you
  - Capillary blood glucose testing kits are readily available and relatively inexpensive, but may provide you with vital information about your athlete
- Usual blood glucose is 4–6 mmol/L though this can increase to 8 mmol/L after meals
- A fasting venous blood glucose of >7 mmol/L is suggestive of diabetes, as is a random blood sugar of >11.1 mmol/L
  - Diagnosis should not be made on the basis of just one blood test especially if there are no specific symptoms
  - Remember the stress response can elevate blood glucose
  - If in doubt, the diagnosis is confirmed using a 2 h glucose tolerance test where blood sugar will be >11.1 mmol/L.

Impaired glucose regulation

This condition is important as it may lead eventually to diabetes, but is managed in the first instance using dietary advice and exercise. It is usually diagnosed where fasting glucose is <7 mmol/L, but oral glucose tolerance test (OGTT) is >7.8 mmol/L, but <11.1 mmol/L.

'Gestational diabetes' encompasses both gestational impaired glucose tolerance and gestational diabetes mellitus. Diagnostic criteria are as above and should be reviewed post-partum.

World Antidoping Agency

Insulin remains a prohibited substance on the World Antidoping Agency WADA's checklist and as such any athlete diagnosed with insulin dependent diabetes must have a therapeutic use exemption certificate competed in accordance with WADA regulations.

Diabetes and exercise

The benefits of exercise on the secondary effects of diabetes such as peripheral and cardiovascular disease is well recognized. It will help in weight loss and promote increased insulin sensitivity. However, glycaemic control can become harder to manage especially in prolonged exercise as glucose stores deplete.

The main aims of diabetic management are to:
- Allow the individual to enjoy life as normally as possible, taking as much responsibility for their disease management as they can. For the athlete, the aims are exactly the same
- The goal is to provide as much education as possible, encouraging the patient to pre-empt the symptoms they are likely to experience such as dehydration and hypoglycaemia by keeping well hydrated and taking enough carbohydrates
- General advice includes taking a carbohydrate snack prior to exercise if the blood sugar level is <5.5 mmol/L. It is a balancing act that may also involve reducing the dose of insulin on days of heavy exercise, and increasing the number of times that the blood glucose is taken
- Self-testing may need to occur, before, during as well as after exercise
- Keeping a stock of easily absorbed carbohydrate readily to hand is vital, and encouraging the athlete to take responsibility for bringing this with them helps to reinforce their autonomy over their disease.

Foot care

Even small wounds affecting the toes can become significant issues with the increased incidence of infection in diabetics. This is compounded by the effects of peripheral vascular disease and neuropathy.
- Regular inspection of footwear, both training and competing can help to minimize the risks of wounds developing
- Good simple foot hygiene and nail care is also vital
- If in doubt refer the athlete to a podiatrist, chiropodist, or back to the diabetic team caring for them.

Diabetes and infection

The aim is to prevent infections from developing, but when they do then insulin requirements will increase. Even in the face of decreased carbohydrate consumption, it is likely you will need to increase the insulin dose.
- Best advice is to be guided by increasing the frequency of monitoring
- Even when appetite is decreased it is important to still try to maintain a reasonable carbohydrate load—even via fluids such as milk and glucose loaded drinks
- Watch out for signs of dehydration especially in the face of vomiting or diarrhoea. Assess for impending ketoacidosis suggested by hyperventilation, tachycardia, and ketotic smell from the athletes breath
- If available test urine for signs of ketones. If in doubt refer to hospital for assessment, intravenous fluid resuscitation, and sliding scale of insulin.

☼ Respiratory

▶▶ For the management of status asthmaticus please refer to 📖 p.94.

Asthma

Asthma is a lower respiratory condition characterized by a triad of:
• Bronchoconstriction
• Increased mucous production
• Mucosal swelling due to inflammation.

This results in shortness of breath, wheeze, and cough, which may be worse at night especially in children. Asthma, like diabetes, is documented to be on the increase and it is highly possible that you will be asked to care for an athlete who suffers from this condition. Early identification of athletes under your care who suffer from asthma is important to ensure you understand their condition prior to any acute episode.
• What inhalers do they take?
• Any previous hospital admissions?
• Any previous intensive therapy unit (ITU) admissions?
• What precipitants are they aware of, particularly non-steroidal anti-inflammatories. Is it exercise induced?
• What is their usual peak flow?

An athlete may present to you with an acute episode of shortness of breath and wheeze heralding a sudden exacerbation or there may be a more gradual deterioration in a patient in whom asthma is either known or suspected, but who has not responded to treatment.

Asthma sufferers participate in sport at all levels up to and including at an elite level. The benefits of exercise should be explained to sufferers who should be reassured and encouraged to participate in an exercise programme.

Exercise induced asthma (EIA)

This condition is characterized by bronchoconstriction induced by histamine release brought about by exercise. The vast majority of patients with asthma will suffer from EIA, although the condition can occur in the general population without a demonstrable diagnosis of asthma at rest.
• In patients reticent to participate in exercise because of the symptoms of EIA, reassurance and a graded exercise programme should be utilized
• Salbutamol should be taken prior to commencing exercise
• An exercise prescription may be useful in such patients to tailor an individual programme.

World Antidoping Agency

Salbutamol and salmeterol are the only two beta–2 agonists not prohibited as long as the manufacturers recommended therapeutic regime is not exceeded.
• Maximum dose of salbutamol is 1600 mcg per 24 h.
• All glucocorticoids are prohibited irrespective of route of administration. See 🔗 www.wada-ama.org.

⚙ Neurological and neuromuscular disorders

Specific medical issues can arise in individuals with neurological and neuromuscular disorders. This chapter aims to cover issues around epilepsy, cerebral palsy, Parkinson's disease, multiple sclerosis, and muscular dystrophy. Cerebrovascular disease and head injury is covered in 📖 Chapter 9 and spinal injury is covered in 📖 Chapter 12.

Epilepsy

Epilepsy is a relatively common condition and is characterized by recurrent unprovoked seizures due to abnormal electrical discharges within the brain. Classified as generalized or partial.
- *Generalized:* here, the epileptic activity involves both halves of the brain. Consciousness is always lost
  - *Grand mal:*
  - Tonic-clonic
  - Clonic
  - Myoclonic
  - *Petit mal:* usually in children. Otherwise known as 'absence' seizures.
- *Partial:* the epileptic activity involves part of the brain
  - Simple—no loss of consciousness
  - Complex—may partly lose consciousness or be unable to remember aspects of the fit.

A partial seizure may progress to a generalized seizure and this is then known as a secondary generalized seizure. Epileptic seizures increase the risk of trauma, fracture, dislocations, burns, and pneumonia due to aspiration. Medical conditions that can predispose to seizures include hypotension, diabetes mellitus, liver, and kidney disease, electrolyte imbalance such as hyper- or hyponatraemia, hypercalcaemia, and alcohol withdrawal.

Main considerations
- Seizure control
- Risk of bodily harm
- Avoidance of seizure precipitating factors. This include stress, sleep deprivation, alcohol, irregular food, and drug intake.

⚠ For the management of seizures notably status epilepticus please refer to 📖 pp.98–99.
- Injury rates for athletes suffering from seizures is not reported as being increased in comparison to athletes who do not suffer from seizures
- However, certain sports may need to be avoided in athletes whose seizure control is poor, such as motorsport
- Caution should always be exercised in the case of known seizure sufferers who should not be allowed to swim without direct supervision and appropriate support
- It is important to be aware of the medications taken by athletes in your care who suffer from seizures, as well as the side effects of the drugs they take

- One of the commonest reasons for seizures in someone already on treatment is sub therapeutic levels of the anticonvulsant +/– poor compliance. It is possible that a decrease in their performance may be related to a side effect of their anticonvulsant treatments.

Cerebral palsy

Cerebral palsy encompasses a group of physical disabilities that appear in infancy or early childhood (see Table 4.1 for a medical classification). The disabilities result from damage to areas in the brain, which can cause loss of balance and posture control, abnormal muscle tone and spinal reflexes, disturbance in sensation, perception, cognition, and communication.

Table 4.1 Medical classification of cerebral palsy

Category	Site of injury	Presentation
Pyramidal	Cortical system	Spastic, hyper-reflexia, 'clasp-knife', hypertonia, prone to contractures
Extrapyramidal	Basal ganglia and cerebellum	Athetosis, ataxia, 'lead-pipe' rigidity, chorea
Mixed	Combination of above	Combination of above

Considerations

- Cardiorespiratory fitness levels can be low in individuals with cerebral palsy, and hence caution may be needed to monitor heart rate, blood pressure (BP) and lactate responses
- Lower peak physiological responses (10–20%)
- Lower mechanical efficiency due to added energy to overcome muscle tonus
- Fatigue and stress can increase symptoms of athetosis and spasticity
- Caution with regards to medications as seizures are common in cerebral palsy, anti-spasmodics, and muscle relaxants used can cause drowsiness and lethargy.

Management

- Physical screening
- Monitor/be aware of dysrhythmias or BP changes
- Be aware of concomitant cognitive, visual, hearing, and speech difficulties
- Do not assume decreased cognitive ability in the presence of drooling or decreased quality of verbal skills.

Parkinson's disease

Parkinson's disease is a chronic progressive disorder involving the extrapyramidal system that regulates muscle reflexes. It is commonly known to consist of a triad of symptoms; rigidity, akinesia (or bradykinesia) and resting tremor. It is thought the reduction of neurotransmitter, dopamine, which is produced in the basal ganglia results in symptoms such as resting tremor, bradykinesia, rigidity, and gait and postural abnormalities.

Relevance to exercise and sport
- Autonomic nervous system dysfunction is common
- Thermal regulation can be difficult to manage with excessive sweating common and fluid losses related to this contributing to dehydration
- Altered heart rate and BP responses
- Movement disorders and muscle rigidity may result in increased oxygen consumption
- Side effect of medications:
  - Levodopa/carbidopa can cause exercise bradycardia, transient peak dose tachycardia and dyskinesia
  - Selegeline can be associated with dyskinesia
  - Some medications are associated with cardiac dysrhythmias
  - Postural Instability can cause balance problems or falls.

Due to paucity of research in this area, general assessment, and management of the athlete with specific consideration to the following is recommended:
- ABC
- Postural issues
- Monitor heart rate and BP
- Cardiac monitor/electrocardiogram (ECG) if suspicion of arrhythmias.

Multiple sclerosis

Multiple sclerosis affects female more than males by a ratio of 2–3:1 and is thought to be an autoimmune condition that affects the myelin sheaths in the neurons in the central nervous system. This results in various symptoms, most notably, spasticity, incoordination, impaired balance, muscle weakness, sensory deficits, autonomic dysfunction of the cardiovascular system, heat sensitivity, and tremor. Exercise in patients with multiple sclerosis (MS) is particularly helpful in maintaining flexibility, cardiovascular fitness as well as helping to prevent secondary complications such as osteoporosis.

Relevance to exercise and sport
- Altered heart rate and BP responses due to cardiovascular autonomic dysfunction
- Heat intolerance
- Sensory loss
- Adequate hydration (urinary frequency, urgency, and incontinence is common, and hence, some individuals may limit fluid intake).

The following general assessment and management is recommended:
- ABC
- Monitor heart rate and BP
- Cardiac monitor/ECG if suspicion of arrhythmias
- Assessment of hydration status—oral/IV fluid as necessary.

Muscular dystrophy

Muscular dystrophy (MD) characterized by progressive muscle weakness, affecting predominantly the skeletal muscles. There are different types of MD namely:
- Duchenne MD
- Becker MD
- Fascio-scapulo-humeral
- Limb girdle
- Myotonic dystrophy.

Depending on the type of dystrophy, symptoms can be mild and progress slowly or progress rapidly causing severe muscle weakness, functional disability, and loss of ability to walk.

The following conditions may occur in individuals with muscular dystrophy:
- Severe muscle weakness, functional disability
- Cognitive delay
- Premature cataracts
- Swallowing problems
- Cardiac conduction block
- Gastrointestinal dysmotility
- Impaired glucose tolerance.

The following general assessment and management is recommended:
- ABC
- Monitor heart rate and BP
- Cardiac monitor/ECG if suspicion of arrhythmias
- Assessment of hydration status—give oral/IV fluid as necessary
- Monitor for muscle cramps. If increasing muscular pain post-exercise especially in the presence of dark urine consider referral to hospital for assessment of possible myoglobinuria secondary to rhabdomyolysis.

✛ Cardiovascular conditions

Cardiovascular disease

Cardiovascular disease in this section will encompass both coronary artery disease (CAD) and conduction disturbances.

Coronary artery disease

CAD encompasses a spectrum of conditions that have the similar pathophysiology of coronary artery narrowing due to atherosclerotic plaques causing myocardial ischaemia.

- Complete obstruction of blood flow to the myocardium leads to myocardial infarction.
- Individuals with CAD are considered to be at high risk of developing life-threatening situations as the cracking of atherosclerotic plaques, with the subsequent formation of platelet aggregation and thrombosis, can cause cardiac events.

Symptoms of CAD include:
- Chest pain
- Palpitations
- Shortness of breath
- Dizziness
- Referred pain to the neck or left arm pain
- Collapse.

Assessment and management of any individuals presenting with suspected coronary artery disease should include the following:
- ABC
- Oxygen via facemask
- Monitor heart rate and BP
- IV access
- *Nitrate:* sublingual if blood pressure is adequate
- Cardiac monitor/ECG
- Call the ambulance
- If there is access to emergency facilities, IV opiate analgesia can be administrated at a titrated dose (by trained medical professional)
- In situations of cardiac arrest, resuscitation guidelines should be followed as described in 📖 p.21.

Conduction disturbances

Conduction disturbances or arrythmias are common in individuals with coronary artery disease, although they can occur in isolation as either congenital or acquired conditions. Among the common arrythmias encountered in this group are:
- Heart blocks, frequent ectopics, and atrial fibrillation
- Supraventricular tachycardia is a common arrythmia found in the younger population, i.e. without CAD
- The danger with all arrythmias is progression to ventricular fibrillation or asystole.

In the event of an arrythmia, assessment and management should be based on identifying the cause and establishing if the arrythmia is new or a known occurrence, which is controlled with treatment. Clinical evaluation of the patient should be as follows:

- ABC
- Oxygen via facemask
- Monitor heart rate and BP
- Cardiac monitor/ECG
- Depending on the arrythmia and its presentation, i.e. new vs. old, controlled vs. uncontrolled, further evaluation, and referral may be necessary
- If in doubt, call the ambulance to transfer to Accident & Emergency (A&E) for further evaluation.

⚠ For the management of supraventricular tachycardias (SVT) arrhythmias see 📖 p.108.

Hypertension

According to the latest British Hypertension Society Guidelines (BHS-IV, 2004), classification of BP levels are as shown in Table 4.2.

Individuals are usually on drug treatment if they have sustained Grade 2 hypertension (>160/100 mmHg) or Grade 1 hypertension with any com-

Table 4.2 Classification of blood pressure levels

Category	Systolic blood pressure (mmHg)	Diastolic blood pressure (mmHg)
Blood pressure		
Optimal	<120	<80
Normal	<130	<85
High normal	130–139	85–89
Hypertension		
Grade 1 (mild)	140–159	90–99
Grade 2 (moderate)	160–179	100–109
Grade 3 (severe)	≥180	≥110
Isolated systolic hypertension		
Grade 1	140–159	<90
Grade 2	≥160	<90

Data from Williams, B., Poulter, N.R., Brown, M.J., et al. (2004). The BHS Guidelines Working Party. British Hypertension Society Guidelines for Hypertension Management—BHS IV: summary. Br Med J **328**: 634–40.

plications. These include target organ damage or if there is an estimated 10-year risk of cardiovascular disease ≥20% despite lifestyle advice.

Considerations on assessment of individuals with hypertension are:
- Heart rate and BP measurement

- BP is usually elevated in individuals that exercise. However, in individuals with hypertension, the absolute level of systolic BP attained during exercise is usually higher due to an elevated baseline level
- Another caution is that these patients maybe on anti-hypertensive treatment; sometimes 2–3 combinations at once. Classes of drugs generally used are angiotensin-converting enzyme inhibitors (ACE-I), angiotensin-II receptor blockers, betablockers, calcium channel blockers, thiazide diuretics, and alphablockers
- Betablockers and to a lesser degree, calcium channel blockers (diltiazem and verapamil) reduce the heart rate response to submaximal and maximal exercise
- Dihydropyridine calcium channel blockers may increase heart rate response to exercise
- Betablockers also reduce the resting BP and the rise of BP from baseline level when exercising
- Alphablockers, calcium channel blockers, and vasodilators may cause post-exertional hypotension
- Diuretics may result in serum potassium abnormalities which may predispose to exercise-induced arrhythmias.

Hence, the following symptoms or signs should prompt further assessment:
- Chest pain
- Dizziness
- Collapse
- Shortness of breath out of proportion to the level of exercise.

When exercising, BP should be maintained below systolic <220 mmHg and diastolic <105 mmHg.

Individuals should not exercise if resting BP is systolic >200 mmHg or diastolic >115 mmHg.

Management
- Stop exercising
- ABC
- Administer oxygen via facemask
- Monitor heart rate and BP
- Cardiac monitor/ECG if there is access
- Depending on the presentation, further assessment, and treatment may be needed with transfer to the hospital if symptoms are not controlled or if further assessment is necessary.

Peripheral vascular disease
Peripheral vascular disease is caused by atherosclerotic lesions in the arteries of the limbs which restrict blood flow distally to the peripheries. A common symptom is intermittent claudication which can present as a cramp or ache in the muscles resulting from exercise. It is typically relieved with rest.

Assessment should include:
- Measures of claudication pain times from history
- Peripheral pulse examination and capillary refill testing (<2 s is normal)
- Ankle–brachial pressure index (ABPI)
- Assess whether coronary artery disease is present.

Management will depend on findings from history and clinical examination:
- ABC
- If distal limb ischaemia is suspected, exercise should be stopped and further referral to a specialist centre or A&E is advised
- Concomitant CAD should be actively sought and treated.

Heart failure

Heart failure refers to the inability of the myocardium to adequately pump blood and hence oxygen and nutrients to the metabolizing tissues in the body. This could be due to systolic dysfunction, diastolic dysfunction, or both.
- Heart failure results in decreased cardiac output during exercise and in severe cases at rest
- There is compensatory ventricular volume overload, mismatch of ventilation to perfusion in the lung, impaired vasodilatation, and renal insufficiency leading to sodium and water retention.

Typically, individuals with heart failure would be on drugs to control their symptoms and progression of disease. These include ACE-I, diuretics, angiotensin receptor blockers or betablockers.

Symptoms of heart failure include:
- Shortness of breath
- Fatigue
- Reduced exercise tolerance
- Peripheral oedema.

Exercise in these individuals also cause different physiological responses:
- Reduced cardiac output due to a drop in ejection fraction and/or stroke volume
- Abnormal blood distribution
- High peripheral resistance
- Exertional hypotension
- Predisposition to arrhythmias.

Hence, assessment and management should include:
- ABC
- Oxygen via face mask
- Heart rate and BP monitoring
- Cardiac monitor/ECG if available
- Intravenous access if not haemodynamically stable
- Consider treatment with diuretics or sublingual GTN if haemodynamically compromised
- Transfer to hospital.

Hypertrophic obstructive cardiomyopathy

Hypertrophic obstructive cardiomyopathy (HOCM) is primarily a disease of the cardiac muscle where the myocardial fibres become hypertrophied and disarrayed. It is thought to be the commonest cause of sudden death in athletes.

Prodromal symptoms may occur in HOCM. However, in many cases, sudden death may the first presentation of this condition. Symptoms and risk factors that should be looked out for are:
• Exertional dyspnoea
• Chest pain
• Palpitations
• Pre-syncope or syncope
• Family history of sudden cardiac death.

In the event of symptoms during exercise in an undiagnosed individual, further investigation will be needed. This includes:
• ECG
• Echocardiography with Doppler
• Further cardiological referral and evaluation if indicated.

In the event of cardiac arrest or collapse, assessment and management should be followed as described in 📖 Chapter 3.

ⓘ Arthritis

Rheumatoid arthritis and ankylosing spondylitis

Rheumatoid arthritis (RA) affects females more commonly than males whilst the opposite is true of ankylosing spondylitis (AS). In RA, onset is usually insidious with stiffness of joints notably in the morning, and increasing pain, and swelling.

- Disease progression eventually leads to deformity of the affected joints commonly affecting the wrist, fingers, and feet
- AS affects the spine and results in back pain
- Rest is appropriate when flare ups of both diseases occur, but exercise is very useful in helping to keep the joints from becoming stiff
- Contact sports should be avoided and swimming is generally accepted as being the exercise most appropriate to minimize impact on joints, whilst providing cardiovascular exercise
- Most athletes with RA will be familiar with the differing medications they will take varying from non-steroidal anti-inflammatories through to steroids and disease modifying anti-rheumatic drugs (DMARDs) such as gold, methotrexate, and penicillamine
- Side effects of these drugs are common and can be debilitating for the patient.

Other issues such as anaemia related to the chronicity of the disease itself or as a direct side effect of the medications may complicate the management of these patients.

- Rheumatoid patients are more likely to suffer from strokes or myocardial infarctions as part of the systemic effects of the inflammation
- Management of most acute presentations is no different in the rheumatoid patient than in the unaffected population
- Exceptions to this include the management of potential cervical spine injuries which can occur with relatively minimal trauma. This should be suspected in anyone with either RA or AS who complains of neck pain after *any* injury
- Both conditions predispose the patient to spinal injury
  - Management differs because the usual technique of spinal immobilization involving lying the patient flat and applying a spinal collar may convert the injury into an unstable one due to the pathological effects of the diseases on the spine
  - The patient should instead lie as flat *as can be tolerated,* a collar applied *if tolerated,* tape, and blocks applied to the each side of the head.

❶ Under no circumstances should anyone with rheumatoid arthritis or ankylosing spondylitis be forced to lie flat wearing a semi-rigid collar if this worsens their symptoms in any way.

⊕ Female athlete triad

The female athlete triad is known to consist of a triad of
- Amenorrhoea
- Osteopenia
- Eating disorders.

Potential complications encountered in this group include collapse due to hypoglycaemia and stress fractures. If stress fractures occur in long bones of the limbs, serious consequences of blood loss may occur.
- Menstrual irregularities can occur due to the combination of exercise intensity and low body weight due to the effect on hypothalamic hormones that control the hypothalamic-gonadal axis
- Delayed menarche, oligomenorrhoea, and amenorrhoea in the years of potential maximal bone mineralization is thought to be associated with lower rate of bone mineral secretion and with increased risks of osteoporotic fractures later in life
- Fracture of the long bones due to normal stresses is a rare, but is a potential complication in the exercising population, especially if there is a history of osteopenia
- However, fractures can occur in all bones where there is impact on exercise, especially due to overuse. Most commonly, this will be bones in the ankle, foot, tibia, and the femur
- General assessment and management will depend on the presentation.
  - Consider ABC
  - Administer oxygen via facemask
  - Beware of cervical spine trauma in the case of a distracting injury. Management with manual in-line stabilization, cervical collar, and spinal board should be followed. This is described further in 📖 Chapter 12
  - IV access
  - Check BP and heart rate
  - Splint the involved area from the joint above to the joint below
  - Check for neurovascular status of the limb involved
  - Ensure systolic BP >80 mmHg. IV fluids may be given to keep systolic BP above this level
  - Transfer to hospital
  - In the case of stress fractures involving the pars interarticularis, it is important to exclude any lower limb neurology.

Further reading

Williams, B., Poulter, N.R., Brown, M.J., et al. (2004). The BHS Guidelines Working Party. British Hypertension Society Guidelines for Hypertension Management—BHS IV: summary. *Br Med J* **328**: 634–40.

Collapse during exercise

Definitions

As well as the common causes of collapse familiar to most medically-trained personnel, athletes are also at risk of collapse from causes that may specifically relate to their particular exercise, such as trauma or extremes of heat:

- Exercise-associated collapse
- Hypothermia
- Heatstroke
- Exercise-associated hyponatraemia
- Cardiac arrest
- Hypoglycaemia
- Anaphylaxis
- Trauma
- Other medical conditions
- Orthopaedic injuries.

Principles of assessment

- Early symptoms and signs may be non-specific and the basic life-support principles of Airway, Breathing, Circulation (A, B, C) must always be attended to first (see 📖 pp. 13–14).
- Loss of consciousness or indeed *any* alteration of mental state (drowsiness, confusion, disorientation, irrational behaviour, aggression, seizures, etc.) suggests a high likelihood of severe hypoglycaemia, hyponatraemia, hyperthermia, or hypothermia.
- Rectal temperature is the only reliable method of assessing core temperature in the field.
- Hydration status is a useful indicator of dehydration, or conversely, hyponatraemia due to fluid overload. For example, from skin turgor, dry mucus membranes, or the inability to spit, through to oedema or puffiness.
- Blood sodium and glucose levels should be checked.
- Site of collapse is an important indicator of severity. Collapse before finishing the event suggests serious illness.

Assessment of the collapsed athlete

- **A:** Airway
- **B:** Breathing
- **C:** Circulation including pulse rate, rhythm, character, and systolic BP
- **D:** Disability or mental status
- **E:** Environment (rectal temperature)
- **F:** Fluid status including change in body weight
- **G:** Blood glucose and sodium
- **H:** History including site of collapse

Accurate diagnosis is vital to ensure that serious causes of collapse are appropriately treated. Except in the case of trauma or cardiac insufficiency, where standard advanced life support (ALS)/advanced trauma life support (ATLS) protocols apply, treatment with intravenous fluids should not be instituted until serum sodium has been checked.

:⚙: Exercise-associated collapse

Exercise-associated collapse (EAC) is the inability to stand or walk unaided as the result of light-headedness, faintness, dizziness, or syncope. EAC is one of the most common reasons for admission to the medical tent at endurance events and classically presents after finishing the event.

EAC is related to postural hypotension that develops upon finishing exercise. Inactivation of the calf muscle pump and subsequent pooling of blood in the legs causes a reduced atrial filling pressure and syncope.

Assessment
- **A:** normal
- **B:** normal
- **C:** postural hypotension (>20 mmHg drop in systolic BP supine to standing). BP and pulse rate normal in supine position
- **D:** usually normal, may have transient loss of consciousness (LOC) during syncope but rapidly resolves in the supine, legs up position
- **E:** ≤39°C
- **F:** normal or dry[1]
- **G:** normal blood glucose and sodium
- **H:** collapse after cessation of exercise.

Treatment
- Place athlete in the Trendelenburg position (supine and head-down, with legs and pelvis elevated)
- Oral fluids.

---

[1] Fluid loss due to sweating, diarrhoea, and vomiting, may contribute to EAC, but there is no evidence that athletes with EAC are any more dehydrated than their non-collapsing counterparts in the same race.

☠ Heatstroke

⚠ Heatstroke can be fatal. The diagnosis of heatstroke is made in anyone with symptoms or signs of organ dysfunction, most commonly altered mental status (including collapse, drowsiness, confusion, etc.) and a rectal temperature >41°C. See Box 5.1 for causes of heat gain and loss.

- Cerebral hyperthermia may lead to hypothalamic failure and loss of thermoregulatory control accelerating the process. Myoglobin release due to rhabdomyolysis can cause renal failure and hyperkalaemia
- Hyperthermia causes suppression of cardiac function leading to reduced cardiac output which may progress through tissue hypoxia, metabolic acidosis to organ dysfunction and multi-system organ failure
- Athletes may remain symptom-free despite rectal temperatures ≤40.5°C. Above this temperature, symptoms tend to occur and an athlete may collapse.

Assessment

- **A:** normal
- **B:** normal, but may be hyperventilating
- **C:** hypotension, tachycardia
- **D:** altered mental state
- **E:** >41°C
- **F:** normal or dry. Sweating may be present, but its absence does not exclude the diagnosis
- **G:** normal blood glucose and sodium
- **H:** presentation may be during or after the event.

Treatment

- Rapid whole body cooling through cold- or ice-water immersion. Alternatively ice-packs to the groin, axillae, and neck may be used
- Close observations and cooling should continue until rectal temperature has reduced, mental status has returned to normal, and cardiovascular function is stable
- Slow recovery or prolonged unconsciousness indicates that hospital admission is required
- Patients may be discharged home from the medical tent if
  - There has been rapid recovery *and*
  - Rectal temperature does not increase in the first hour after cessation of active cooling.

Box 5.1 Heat gain and loss in exercise

Heat gain
- *Endogenous:* muscle activity and metabolism
- *Exogenous:* environmental

Heat loss in exercise
- In low environmental temperatures (below body temperature), heat is lost through convection and radiation from the skin, with some contribution from conduction. During exercise and when environmental temperature ≥ body temperature sweating allows much more effective heat loss through evaporation.
- In humid conditions however, evaporation is reduced and cooling becomes less effective. An athlete may be unable to lose heat during exercise in high temperature and high humidity environments and so begin to overheat, even in relatively short-distance races and in seemingly cool conditions. Exercise in such situations becomes dangerous.
- The wet bulb globe temperature (WBGT) index takes into account the humidity as well as solar and ground radiation in combination with air temperature and wind speed. The American College of Sports Medicine has produced guidelines for the amount of exercise that can be safely carried out in hot conditions based on the WBGT.

☠ Hypothermia

Hypothermia is defined by a core temperature <35°C. It occurs when body heat losses exceeds heat generated.

- Peripheral sensory nerves relay information on temperature to central receptors in the hypothalamus, which responds by stimulating shivering to generate body heat
- The receptors in the skin are more sensitive to the rate of change in temperature than the actual temperature
- A rapid drop in temperature, for example falling into cold water, is felt more acutely than a slow decrease
- Thus a gradual drop in temperature may not be accompanied by a sense of cold and shivering may not be initiated.

⚠ The athlete may therefore not be aware of the cold.

Athletes are at risk of hypothermia when they are unable to generate enough body heat to keep the body warm. This may occur in relatively warm temperatures!

Risk factors

- *Exhaustion:* slow moving, unable to generate body heat through activity
- Hypoglycaemia impairs shivering
- Inadequate clothing or protective equipment
- *Rain:* increases heat loss through convection
- *Cold wind:* wind chill factor effectively reduces the temperature and increases heat loss through evaporation
- *Accident or injury:* leaving athlete exposed
- *Immersion in cold water:* much greater heat loss through convection.

Physiological effects

- Peripheral vasoconstriction to reduce body heat losses and to protect core temperature. This underlines the importance of measurement of core body temperature (with a rectal thermometer) rather than peripheral temperature (oral, tympanic, or axillae)
- Reduced cardiac output. Myocardial depression and impaired electrical conduction combined with reduced circulating volume as a result of fluid loss from sweating and respiration during exercise
- Cardiac arrhythmias. Impaired electrical conduction leading to decreased heart rate initially with prolonged segments on electrocardiogram (ECG). ST segment J-waves may be evident, suggesting hypothermia. Atrial fibrillation (AF) and ventricular fibrillation (VF) may occur. AF may settle with rewarming
- Hyperventilation is a cold-induced reflex and may exacerbate dehydration and heat loss.

Neurological changes

- Involuntary shivering initially, later muscle rigidity
- Hyper-reflexia initially, diminished or absent reflexes in severe hypothermia

- Dysarthria, slow reaction time, impaired co-ordination, and delayed cerebration due to delayed nerve conduction
- Amnesia progressing through confusion and drowsiness to loss of consciousness.

Assessment of hypothermia

Classified into mild, moderate, and severe hypothermia dependent upon symptoms and temperature, although symptoms may vary from person to person. (Table 5.1)

Table 5.1 Assessment of hypothermia

	Mild	Moderate	Severe
A	Normal	Normal, Can develop bronchospasm	Normal, Can develop pulmonary oedema
B	Tachypnoea	Tachypnoea	Hypoventilation
C	Tachycardia	Tachycardia	Hypotension, bradycardia, arrhythmias (including VF), asystole
D	Subjective feeling of cold, shivering, Amnesia, dysarthria, apathy, signs of withdrawal	Reduced shivering, Fatigue, drowsiness, confusion, poor judgment	Muscle rigidity Inappropriate behaviour, reduced level of consciousness
E	33–35°C, cold conditions, rain, and/or wind	31–32°C, cold conditions, rain, and/or wind	<3°C, cold conditions, rain, and/or wind
F	Urinary urgency*	Dehydration	Dehydration
G	Normal	Normal to low	Normal to low
H	During or after event, inadequate clothing or protection, accident or injury, immersion		

*Peripheral vasoconstriction temporarily induces an increase in central blood volume, which causes a cold diuresis, contributing to dehydration.

Treatment of hypothermia

Mild

Active rewarming: warm clothes, warm sweet drink, hot packs to torso, or hot tub.

Moderate

- *Passive rewarming only in the field setting*: remove from cold environment, remove wet clothes, insulate
- *Transfer to hospital for active rewarming*: continual cardiovascular monitoring for hypotension and arrhythmias.

Severe
- Passive rewarming only in the field setting, *but* handle the patient as little as possible to avoid risk of precipitating ventricular fibrillation
- Transfer to intensive care for active rewarming.

Further notes
- Space blankets do not prevent further heat loss. In established hypothermia, continuing heat loss is primarily through convection, not radiation
- Avoid further exercise. Glycogen depletion through exercise will prevent shivering
- Apply hot packs to torso only, as peripheral rewarming increases peripheral blood flow reducing central blood volume. This may lead to cardiovascular collapse. Hot tubs provide hydrostatic support so help to maintain blood pressure
- Remove a hypothermic patient from cold water in the horizontal position. Loss of hydrostatic pressure from the water may precipitate hypotension and cardiovascular collapse.

❶ At very low temperatures, signs of life may be difficult to detect. Death cannot be determined until after rewarming.

A person is not dead until 'warm and dead'.

☼ Exercise-associated hyponatraemia

Exercise-associated hyponatraemia (EAH) is a rare, but preventable cause of death in endurance exercise.

- EAH should be considered a possible diagnosis in anyone with altered mental status including seizures or unconsciousness during or after an endurance event. Core temperature will be normal. Seizures may also be the initial presentation
- EAH is a dilutional hyponatraemia caused by fluid intake in excess of body fluid losses during or in the first 24 h after exercise. Inappropriate anti-diuretic hormone (ADH) release during exercise may be an additional contributing factor
- Relative hyponatraemia in the vascular compartment causes an osmotic fluid shift into adjacent tissues, which manifests itself as puffiness and oedema peripherally, but centrally as cerebral and pulmonary oedema
- Early signs and symptoms are non-specific (nausea, vomiting, puffiness, bloating) and may be confused with those of dehydration. In a similar fashion, lack of urination, more commonly attributed to dehydration, may be a sign of ongoing renal impairment due to ADH
- More severe cases may develop signs of central nervous system dysfunction such as confusion, aggression, seizure, stupor, or coma.

Pulmonary and cerebral oedema, if untreated, will cause death.

Risk factors

- ♂>♀
- Long distance event (usually >4 hr)
- Consumption of more than 3 L of fluid
- Weight gain during the race
- Low body mass index
- Slow race pace.

Assessment

- **A:** normal
- **B:** normal, but tachypnoea and hypoxia may develop with pulmonary oedema
- **C:** normal, well filled
- **D:** normal in early EAH, altered mental state as severity increases
- **E:** ≤39°C
- **F:** normal or overloaded.[1] A history of copious fluid consumption during or after the event may be available, but cannot be relied upon, especially if confused. Little or no urination suggests renal dysfunction
- **G:** serum sodium <135 mmol/L. Normal glucose
- **H:** collapse during or up to 24 h after the event.

---

1 Observe for facial and peripheral puffiness or oedema. Also look for tight rings, watchstraps, socks, etc.

Treatment

- Alert and orientated individuals and sodium <135mmol/L (mild-moderate EAH):
  - Give salty snacks or salty broth
  - Observe closely
  - No oral fluids until onset of urination
- Any evidence of altered mental state or pulmonary oedema and sodium <135mmol/L (severe EAH):
  - Administer oxygen
  - Administer 100 mL IV bolus of 3% salt which may be repeated up to 3 times at 10-min intervals if required
- Hypotonic or isotonic solutions (including 0.9% salt) are contra-indicated
- May require hospital admission to receive further treatment including ventilatory support, especially if slow to improve.

Notes

Weight gain during exercise is a valid marker of fluid overload. Runners should expect to lose up to 2% body weight over the course of a marathon due to carbohydrate/substrate utilization.

- Therefore, even neutral weight balance and weight loss <2% are indicators of fluid overload
- Urgent sodium level must be obtained and catheterization may be undertaken to aid assessment of renal function.

Prevention

- Avoid excessive drinking during exercise. Encourage ad libitum drinking—rely on your thirst telling you when to drink. It is a very sophisticated and accurate mechanism
- Weigh athletes before and after training runs in different weather conditions drinking the fluids available at the race in order to better understand how their body reacts to fluid. Neutral weight balance or weight gain on runs >21 miles suggests they have drunk too much
- Avoid excessive drinking after exercise. The risk of EAH remains present for several hours afterwards
- Sodium-containing sports drinks do not prevent EAH if they are consumed excessively. They too are hypotonic or isotonic and will contribute to the inherent dilution of EAH.

Further reading

Almond, C.S., Shin, A.Y., Fortescue, E.B., et al. (2005). Hyponatremia among runners in the Boston Marathon. *N Engl J Med* **352**: 1550–6.

Armstrong, L.E., Casa, D.J., Millard-Stafford, M., et al. (2007). American College of Sports Medicine position stand. Exertional heat illness during training and competition. *Med Sci Sports Exer* **39**(3): 556–72.

Castellani, J.W., Young, A.J., Ducharme, M.B., et al. (2006). American College of Sports Medicine position stand. Prevention of cold injuries during exercise. *Med Sci.Sports Exer* **38**(11): 2012–29.

Hew-Butler, T., Ayus, J.C., Kipps, C., et al. (2007). Statement of the Second International Exercise-Associated Hyponatremia Consensus Development Conference, New Zealand. *Clin J Sport Med* **18**(2): 111–21.

Holtzhausen, L.M., Noakes, T.D., Kroning, B., et al. (1994). Clinical and biochemical characteristics of collapsed ultra-marathon runners. *Med Sci Sports Exer* **26**(9): 1095–101.

Noakes, T. (2001). Exercise in the heat. In: Bruckner, P., Khan, K. (eds) *Clinical Sports Medicine*, 2nd edn. Sydney: McGraw-Hill Australia Pty Ltd. 798–806.

Noakes, T. (2001). Exercise in the cold. In: Bruckner, P., Khan, K. (eds) *Clinical Sports Medicine*, 2nd edn. Sydney: McGraw-Hill Australia Pty Ltd, 807–15.

Roberts, W.O. (1994). Assessing core temperature in collapsed athletes: what's the best method? *Physician Sportsmed.* **22**(8):49–55.

Roberts, W.O. (2007). Exercise-associated collapse care matrix in the marathon. *Sports Med* **37**(4–5): 431–33.

Speedy, D.B., Noakes, T., Holtzhausen, L.M. (2005). Exercise associated collapse: postural hypotension, or something deadlier? *Physic Sportsmed* **31**(3): 23–9.

Altitude sickness

Altitude sickness

What goes up must come down

Barometric pressure falls linearly with increasing altitude. The oxygen concentration of air remains constant at 21%, regardless of altitude. Consequently, the partial pressure of oxygen in ambient air reduces proportionately with increasing altitude (Fig. 6.1). It is this hypobaric hypoxia that leads to the spectrum of medical conditions commonly referred to as altitude sickness.

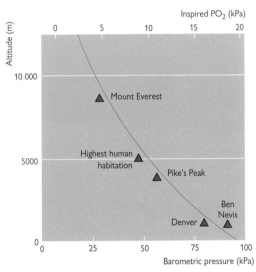

Fig. 6.1 The effect of altitude on the partial pressure of oxygen. Reproduced from Johnson et al., *Oxford Handbook of Expedition and Wilderness Medicine*, 2008, with permission from Oxford University Press.

Definition of altitude

- *High altitude:* 1500–3500 m
- *Very high altitude:* 3500–5500 m
- *Extreme altitude:* above 5500 m.

Altitude sickness

Altitude sickness is an umbrella term used to describe the following three acute conditions:

- Acute mountain sickness (AMS) occurs in 50–70% of those ascending to above 3500 m
- High altitude cerebral oedema (HACE) occurs in around 1% of people ascending to 4000–5500 m

- High altitude pulmonary oedema (HAPE) occurs in around 2% ascending to 4000–5500 m.

AMS and HACE are thought to involve the same cerebral pathology and represent the mild and life-threatening ends of the spectrum, respectively. HAPE, a pulmonary illness, may present independent of AMS. It is important to highlight. However, all three conditions manifest from the same hypoxic insult and there is therefore frequent concurrence with significant clinical overlap.

Normal physiology in response to altitude

In order to survive at altitude the body must acclimatize by employing a multi-system response:

- *Respiratory:* increased minute ventilation to improve oxygenation (known as the hypoxic ventilatory response). Consequent lowering of $PaCO_2$ results in a respiratory alkalosis
- *Renal:* increased excretion of bicarbonate ions and retention of H^+ ions compensates the development of alkalosis and allows further increases in ventilation. This adaptation explains the polyuria often experienced at altitude
- *Cardiovascular:* increased heart rate, cardiac output, and vasoconstriction of pulmonary vasculature attempt to improve gaseous exchange and delivery of oxygenated blood to tissues
- *Haematological:* in response to the low PaO_2 there is increased hemoglobin production to improve the oxygen-carrying capacity of the blood
- *Neurological:* cerebral blood flow has been shown to increase significantly during ascent to high altitude.

Prevention

- Avoid rapid ascension to altitudes above 2000–2500 m
- Ascend slowly with stops at intermediate altitudes
- Avoid vigorous exercise on the first few days of arrival
- Acetazolamide (125 mg–250 mg twice daily (bd)) beginning 48 hr before ascent to altitude and continued for 5 days has been shown to be beneficial in prevention of symptoms.

Differential diagnoses (Table 6.1)

Table 6.1 Differential diagnoses of altitude sickness

Acute mountain sickness	High altitude pulmonary oedema
Dehydration	Pulmonary embolus
Hypoglycaemia	Infection
Hypothermia	Myocardial infarction
Hyponatraemia	
Cerebral infection	
Space occupying lesion	
Stroke	

☼ Acute mountain sickness

More than half of people ascending to an altitude of 3500 m will suffe
AMS. Although often not an emergency in itself it is imperative to be able
to recognize and manage AMS appropriately to avoid life-threatening
sequelae, such as HACE/HAPE.

Typical onset
- Altitudes between 2500–3500 m (high altitude)
- Within 4–24 hr of ascent to altitude.

Symptoms
See Table 6.2.
  Headache (frontal/generalized) plus at least one of:
- Nausea
- Vomiting
- Dizziness
- Lethargy/listlessness
- Sleep disturbance.

Table 6.2 Lake Louise Symptom Score for AMS. A score of 3–5
is considered diagnostic of mild/moderate AMS. A score >6 is
diagnostic of severe AMS

Symptoms	Severity	Points
Headache	No headache	0
	Mild headache	1
	Moderate headache	2
	Severe headache, incapacitating	3
Gastrointestinal	No gastrointestinal symptoms	0
	Poor appetite or nausea	1
	Moderate nausea or vomiting	2
	Severe nausea or vomiting	3
Fatigue and/or weakness	Not tired or weak	0
	Mild fatigue/weakness	1
	Moderate fatigue/weakness	2
	Severe fatigue/weakness, incapacitating	3
Dizziness/ lightheadedness	Not dizzy	0
	Mild dizziness	1
	Moderate dizziness	2
	Severe dizziness, incapacitating	3

Table 6.2 *Continued*

Symptoms	Severity	Points
Difficulty of sleeping	Slept as well as usual	0
	Did not sleep as well as usual	1
	Woke up many times, poor night's sleep	2
	Unable sleep	3

Reproduced from UIAA Medical Commission Consensus Statement No. 2: Emergency Field Management of Acute Medical Sickness, High Altitude Pulmonary Oedema, and High Altitude Cerebral Oedema, 2009, with permission from the International Climbing and Mountain Federation (UIAA)

Management (mild/moderate) (see Fig. 6.2)

- Rest and avoid further ascent
- Ensure patient remains well hydrated
- Symptomatic treatment (anti-emetics, simple analgesia), although it is usually self-limiting
- Descend if symptoms worsen or do not improve within 24 hr
- Only consider continuing ascent once patient is symptom free.

Management (severe)

- Rest
- Descend (at least 500 m)
- Symptomatic treatment (anti-emetics, simple analgesia)
- Acetazolamide (250 mg bd)
- Consider dexamethasone (8 mg, then 4 mg every 6 hr).

If descent is not possible

- Oxygen
- Portable hyperbaric chamber (e.g. Gamow Bag).

Note: distinguishing severe AMS and HACE can be difficult. If in doubt, treat as HACE.

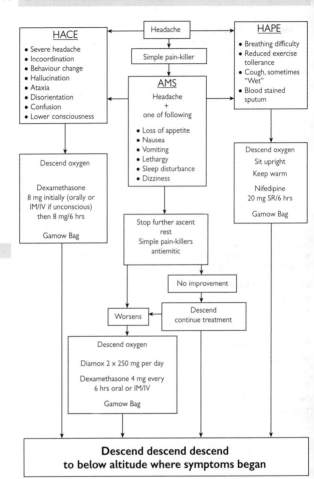

Fig. 6.2 Management flow chart for altitude sickness. Reproduced from UIAA Medical Commission Consensus Statement No. 2: Emergency Field Management of Acute Medical Sickness, High Altitude Pulmonary Oedema, and High Altitude Cerebral Oedema, 2009, with permission from the International Climbing and Mountain Federation (UIAA).

☠ High altitude cerebral oedema

HACE represents the extreme of AMS and is a rare and life threatening emergency. It is a clinical diagnosis defined by the development of altered mental status and/or ataxia in a patient with AMS (or HAPE).

Typical onset

- Altitudes between 4000 and 5500 m (very high altitude)
- 1–3 days after ascent to altitude.

Symptoms/signs

- Headache refractory to simple analgesics
- Nausea
- Vomiting
- Dizziness
- Ataxia (heel-to-toe walking is a sensitive field test)
- Cognitive impairment, e.g. confusion, irrational behaviour
- Coma.

Management (Fig. 6.2)

- Organize urgent descent or evacuation
- Portable hyperbaric chamber if descent not possible
- Oxygen
- Dexamethasone (8 mg, then 4–8 mg every 6 hr)
- Acetazolamide (250 mg bd)
- If symptoms do not improve with the above consider alternative diagnoses (see 📖 Table 6.2).

☼: High altitude pulmonary oedema

HAPE is the most common cause of death from altitude-related illness.

Typical onset
- Altitudes between 4000 and 5500 m (very high altitude)
- 1–3 days after ascent to altitude (typically the 2nd night).

Symptoms/signs
- Worsening dyspnoea on exertion, becoming symptomatic at rest
- Tachypnoea
- Persistent cough, becoming productive of frothy/bloody sputum
- Severe fatigue and exercise intolerance
- Crackles/wheeze in at least one lung field
- Tachycardia
- Cyanosis
- Fever (often leading to misdiagnosis of chest infection).

Management (Fig. 6.2)
- Increasing oxygenation is the highest priority in HAPE
- Organize urgent descent or evacuation
- Use a portable hyperbaric chamber if descent not possible
- Oxygen
- Keep upper body upright to minimize effects of oedema
- Avoid exertion (raises pulmonary arterial pressure)
- Prevent cold/hypothermia (raises pulmonary arterial pressure)
- Nifedipine slow release:
  - 20 mg, repeated every 6–8 hr if necessary
  - Effects should be evident after 15 min
- Acetazolamide (250 mg bd)
- Salmeterol (can help clearance of alveolar fluid)
- The use of diuretics is not beneficial in the treatment of HAPE
- If symptoms do not improve consider alternative diagnoses
  (see 🕮 Table 6.2).

Note: if you are unsure whether someone is suffering HAPE or HACE, then treat empirically (severe HAPE can often trigger HACE) by organizing descent (or hyperbaric chamber), oxygen, dexamethasone, nifedipine, and acetazolamide.

Pathophysiology

The exact pathophysiology involved in altitude sickness remains very much unclear.

- *AMS/HACE:* hypoxaemia initiates a vasodilatory response that results in increased cerebral blood flow. The increased capillary pressure (possibly combined with worsened capillary permeability) eventually leads to the development of cerebral oedema.
- *HAPE:* vasoconstriction of the pulmonary circulation following hypoxic insult leads to pulmonary hypertension. This is responsible for the development of the non-cardiogenic, hydrostatic pulmonary oedema seen in HAPE.

Drugs

Acetazolamide (Diamox®)

- Carbonic anhydrase inhibitor
- Accelerates acclimatization by promoting bicarbonate diuresis and providing respiratory stimulus (see 📖 p.67)
- It does not mask the symptoms of altitude sickness
- Often used prophylactically if sufficient acclimatization will not be possible or person is at high risk of developing AMS:
  - Start 1 day before ascending to altitude
  - Continue for 2 days once at maximum altitude
- *Side effects:* tingling in extremities, altered taste, polyuria.

Dexamethasone

- Potent steroid
- Improves cerebral oedema
- Drug treatment of choice in HACE/AMS
- Does not accelerate acclimatization (unlike acetazolamide)
- *Can mask AMS:* do *not* ascend whilst taking dexamethasone
- *Side effects:* rebound AMS if suddenly withdrawn, mood changes, hyperglycaemia, dyspepsia.

Nifedipine

- Calcium-channel blocker
- Reduces pulmonary artery pressure
- Drug treatment of choice in HAPE (variable results)
- May be prescribed for prophylaxis of HAPE in recurrent sufferers
- *Side effects:* reflex tachycardia, hypotension.

Who is at risk?

Everyone is at risk of developing altitude sickness regardless of sex, age, fitness level, and race; it is notoriously unpredictable.

Risk factors for altitude sickness
- Previous history of altitude sickness (most relevant)
- Fast ascent to high altitude
- Higher altitude
- Dehydration
- Strenuous exercise at altitude (most relevant to HAPE)
- Ignoring early symptoms
- Gaining more than 300–500 m in sleeping altitude per day (relevant at altitudes greater than 3000 m)
- Some research shows young people (<50 years old) and men may be more susceptible (though this may be a reflection of the more aggressive ascent profiles used by these groups)
- Removal/destruction of carotid body (e.g. due to surgery or radiotherapy) will affect the ability to initiate an hypoxic ventilatory response and hence acclimatization
- Pre-existing pulmonary hypertension will increase risk of HAPE.

Note: smoking, hypertension, coronary artery disease (CAD), asthma, and mild chronic obstruction pulmonary disease do not appear to affect susceptibility to high-altitude illness. Physical fitness is not protective.

Key learning points
- Consider everyone to be at risk of altitude sickness
- There is significant individual variation in clinical presentation
- Illness at altitude is altitude sickness until proven otherwise
- Have a low threshold to diagnose and treat as HACE or HAPE
- Do not ascend with symptoms of AMS
- Descend urgently if symptoms worsen or HACE/HAPE develop
- Descent is the key to treatment; other measures (drugs, hyperbaric chambers) are intervening measures that buy you time
- Acetazolamide does not mask symptoms
- Never ascend whilst on dexamethasone
- If symptoms do not improve on descent, review your diagnosis
- Adopt a conservative ascent profile to prevent altitude sickness.

Further reading

Clarke, C. (2006). Acute mountain sickness: medical problems associated with acute and subacute exposure to hypobaric hypoxia. *Postgrad Med J* **82**: 748–53.

Hacket, P.H., Roach, R. (2001). High altitude illness. *N Engl J Med* **345**: 107–14.

UIAA Medical Commission (2008). *Consensus Statement*. International Climbing and Mountain Federation (UIAA). Bern, 1–16.

UIAA Mountain Medical Centre Information sheets (2002).

Himalayan Mountain Rescue Association. Available at: www.himalayanrescue.org.

Wilderness Medical Society. Available at: www.wms.org.

International Climbing and Mountain Federation. Available at: www.theuiaa.org.

British Mountaineering Council. Available at: www.thebmc.co.uk.

MEDEX. Available at: www.medex.org.uk.

Sudden cardiac death in sport

Epidemiology

Sudden death in sport, although rare, is absolutely devastating for the family of the athlete. It can also have a negative impact on the sport itself. It is always a concern for a doctor covering any sporting event.

Screening may identify those at risk, but also raises the possibility of identifying and excluding unaffected athletes. It remains controversial.

Doctors are often asked to 'screen' participants to ensure they are fit to participate.

- Much of the current data is from the USA (collegiate sport—basketball, swimming, track, field, American football, and soccer) or from Northern Italy
- More commonly occurs in the over 35 years age group due to ischaemic heart disease
- Abnormal echocardiogram findings of hypertrophic cardiomyopathy are seen in up to 1/500 athletes as part of routine screening. The actual reported prevalence of sudden cardiac death varies widely between 1 in 27,000 to 1 in 300,000, in the under 35 years age group. (This may be underreported due to media—rather than post mortem—reports.)
- In the under 35 years age group, sudden death is more common in black teenage males
- There is a geographical variation in causative pathology in various parts of the world, e.g. hypertrophic cardiomyopathy is most common in North America, whereas arrythmogenic right ventricular dysplasia is more prevalent in Italy.

Aetiology

In the over 35's, ischaemic heart disease is, by far, the commonest cause. There are a number of causes in under 35's.

Congenital

Hypertrophic cardiomyopathy (HOCM)
- Leading cause of death in 36% of cases
- Predisposition to supraventricular and ventricular arrhythmias
- *Clinical signs:*
  - Jerky pulse
  - Double apex beat
  - Fourth heart sound
  - Ejection systolic murmur
  - Abnormal ECG in 90%
  - Characteristic echocardiograph features
- *Adverse prognostic signs:*
  - Family history sudden death
  - Autosomal dominance inheritance
  - Ventricular tachycardia (VT) episodes
  - Young age of symptom onset

Idiopathic concentric left ventricle (LV) hypertrophy
- Associated with athletic training
- Increased incidence in black athletes
- ECHO changes reduce with deconditioning over 6 month period.

Anomalous coronary artery origins
Left coronary travels between aorta and pulmonary trunk from right coronary sinus, compressed frequently at high heart rates—fall in coronary perfusion pressure—leading to chest pain, syncope, or sudden death.
- *Investigations:*
  - Changes may be found on resting electrocardiogram (ECG)
  - Stress ECG testing
  - Coronary angiography

Long QT
- QT prolonged to more than 0.44 s corrected for heart rate
  - Increased risk ventricular arrhythmias
  - Episodes associated with stress and exercise
  - Treated with betablockers, sympathectomies, or pacemakers

Wolff-Parkinson White
- Short PR interval—less than 0.12 s
- Delta wave on ECG gives appearance of wide QRS
- Accessory pathways lead to atrial arrhythmias and possible VF
- Surgical ablation of the pathway maybe required

Arrhythmnogenic right ventricular dysplasia

- Right ventricular cardiomyopathy
- Leads to ventricular arrhythmias
- High incidence in Northern Italy.

Aortic rupture

- Marfan syndrome is a connective tissue derangement leading to increased incidence of aortic dissection and rupture
  - Congenital—autosomal dominant
  - Musculoskeletal, ocular, and cardiovascular abnormalities
  - Patients appear tall with long slender limbs, high arched palette, and visual problems

Valvular disease

Can be congenital, acquired, or degenerative.

- Aortic stenosis
  - Management depends on presence of symptoms: chest pain, breathlessness, syncope
  - If moderate then restriction of sporting activity suggested.

Acquired

Post-viral cardiomyopathy

- Viral illness leading to lymphocytic infiltration of the heart muscle, leading to reduction of cardiac function and potential arrhythmias
- Athletes with a pyrexia should be rested

Ischaemic heart disease

- Resting ECG may not show any abnormality
- Stress ECG, cardiac computed tomography (CT), or cardiac angiography investigations of choice.

Presentation

The presentation of a patient with risk factors for sudden cardiac death maybe subtle.

Over 35-year-olds

In the over 35-years-old age group, the classical presentation of exertional angina may not be present, but should always be asked about in a patient prior to undertaking exercise. Other risk factors for ischaemic heart disease should be sought including:

- Diabetes
- Smoking
- Hypercholesterolaemia
- Family history
- Hypertension
- Previous history of ischaemia, valvular, or structural heart disease.

The resting ECG may not be helpful and more specific tests are often required to exclude the possibility of hidden cardiac disease.

Under 35-year-olds

In this age group symptoms of syncope, chest pain, unexplained shortness of breath, palpitations, or dizziness should always be taken seriously and a full assessment performed which should include:

- A full history
- A cardio-respiratory clinical examination
- ECG
- Then an echocardiograph if indicated or the symptoms are recurrent.

Sometimes a coach may identify an athlete as being overly 'tired' or having reduced exercise tolerance. Although vague, such subtle symptoms should also be considered as potentially originating from an occult cardiac cause. The examination for a potential cardiac cause should be included as part of the investigation of this patient.

Screening

Veneto experience in northern Italy
- Screen every competitive athlete in general population at school age
- Abnormality means exclusion from sport
- Based on 25 years of data
- 90% reduction in death from hypertrophic cardiomyopathy (HCM)
- Not repeated elsewhere, e.g. Northern Europe.

Screening tools
- *Family history:* good for autosomal dominant HCM/ischaemic heart disease (IHD)
- *Symptoms and sign:* the majority of deaths have no preceding signs or symptoms. However, any should be investigated fully
- *ECG:*
  - International Olympic Committee & European Heart Association recommend ECG screening, although the American Heart Association do not
  - ECG changes are sometimes difficult to interpret due the 'normal' changes associated with the athletic heart. If there is any doubt then a cardiology expert opinion should be sought to report the ECG
  - 2010 European ECG criteria are associated with improved specificity, but preserved sensitivity than 2005 criteria
- *Other—echocardiogram (echo)/magnetic resonance imaging (MRI):*
  - Less useful as screening tool for large population
  - 1 in 500 athletes screened will have an abnormal ECHO but it should be remembered that the prevalence of SCD is variably reported
  - Hypertrophied 'athletic heart' can mimic HCM on echocardiogram (ECHO).

The outcome of a screening programme may have significant effects with ethical issues affecting both athlete and clinician. There are potential insurance, mortgage, and employment implications for the athlete of having a diagnosis made, even though there is a very small risk of death.

Screening for a team
Advantages
- Possibly easier to fund
- Easier to control population group
- Access to specialist sports cardiology opinions
- Easier access to more advanced investigations
- Perceived by public and athletes that screening will reduce/prevent on-field sudden cardiac death (SCD).

Disadvantages
- Cardiac screening will not prevent all on-field SCD due to some of the unscreenable acquired causes (e.g. IHD/post-viral myocarditis/variable penetrance of HCM)
- Time-intensive as informed consent is required

- *Ethical issues:*
  - A player may not want to be screened
  - A player may wish to ignore the advice given following the screening programme
  - Informed consent is required.

2010 Recommendations for interpretation of 12-lead electrocardiogram in the athlete (Table 7.1)

Table 7.1 Classification of abnormalities of the athlete's electrocardiogram

Group 1: Common and training-related ECG changes	Group 2: Uncommon and training-unrelated ECG changes
Sinus bradycardia	T-wave inversion
First-degree AV block	ST-segment depression
Incomplete RBBB*	Pathological Q-waves
Early repolarization	Left atrial enlargement
Isolated QRS voltage criteria for left ventricular hypertrophy	Left-axis deviation/left anterior hemiblock
	Right-axis deviation/left posterior hemiblock
	Right ventricular hypertrophy
	Ventricular pre-excitation
	Complete LBBB or RBBB*
	Long- or short-QT interval
	Brugada-like early repolarization

* RBBB, right bundle branch block; LBBB, left bundle branch block.

Reproduced from Corrado D, Pellicia A et al.Recommendations for interpretation of 12-lead electrocardiogram in the athlete, *European Heart Journal*, 2010, **31**(2): pp. 243–59, by permission of European Society of Cardiology.

☠ Management

Sudden cardiac death

Anticipation of an event is important. Access to a defibrillator and other equipment to aid basic life support (BLS) is vital.

Regular updates and simulation training should be undertaken by any health care professional involved in sport. Preparation for a cardiac event on the field of play, or in the crowd, should be anticipated and planned for.

The minimum requirements for equipment would include:
- Defibrillator, regularly serviced and up to date with latest support software
- Pocket ventilation device
- Airway support devices, e.g. oropharyngeal airway.

Other equipment will depend on the expertize of the heath care professional. (see 📖 p.18).
- The approach should be the same as for any 'collapsed' patient, although early defibrillation is important as the most likely arrhythmia will be ventricular in origin
- Unfortunately, survival to discharge in the under 35-years athletic group is still poor, despite high quality cardiopulmonary resuscitation (CPR) and early defibrillation. This may possibly be due to the genetic nature of serious cardiac pathology.

Prevention

Exercising and viral illness

- If pyrexial, avoid strenuous exercise
- If apyrexial and symptoms in one system only (e.g. coryza), normal activity is permitted
- If apyrexial and symptoms in two or more systems (e.g. coryza, cough, myalgia), no 'vigorous' activity is permitted.

Pre-sudden cardiac death pathology and treatments

- *Hypertrophic cardiomyopathy:*
  - Calcium antagonists/beta blockers
  - Septal myectomy
  - Implantable defibrillator
- *Anomalous coronary artery origins:* surgical re-implantation
- *Ion channelopathies:*
  - Wolff–Parkinson–White syndrome—radiofrequency ablation of ac-cessory pathways
  - Long Q–T syndrome—drugs, genetic counselling, implantable defibrillators.

Further reading

Corrado, D., Basso, C., Schiavon, M., et al. (1998). Screening for hypertrophic cardiomyopathy in young athletes. *N Engl J Med* **339**(6): 364–9.

Corrado, D., Basso, C., Schiavon, M., et al. (2008). Pre-participation screening of young athletes fo prevention of SCD. *J Am Coll Cardiol* **52**(24): 1981–9.

Corrado, D., Pelliccia, A., Bjørnstad, H.H., et al. (2005). Cardiovascular preparticipation screening of young competitive athletes for prevention of sudden death: proposal for a common Euro-pean protocol. *Eur Heart J* 26: 516–24.

Corrado, D., Pellicia, A., Heidbuchel, H., et al. (2010). Recommendations for interpretation of 12-lead electrocardiogram in the athlete. *Eur Heart J* **31**(2): 243–59.

Drezner, J.A. (2008). Contemporary approaches to the identification of athletes at risk for sudden cardiac death. *Curr Opin Cardiol* **23**(5): 494–501.

Eckart, R.E., Scoville, S.L., Campbell, C.L., et al. (2004). Sudden death in young adults: a 25-year review of autopsies in military recruits. *Ann Intern Med* **141**(11): 829–34.

Harmon, K.G., Irfan, M.A., Klosner, D., et al. (2011). Incidence of cardiac death in National Collegiate Athletic Association athletes. *Circulation* **123**: 1594–600.

Maron, B.J., Doerer, J.J., Haas, T.S., et al. (2009). Sudden deaths in young competitive athletes: analysis of 1866 deaths in the United States. *Circulation*, **119**(8): 1085–92.

Maron, B.J., Pelliccia, A., Spataro, A., et al. (1993). Reduction in left ventricular wall thickness after deconditioning in highly trained Olympic athletes. *Br Heart J* **69**: 125–8.

Maron, B.J., Thompson, P.D., Ackerman, M.J., et al. (2007). Recommendations and considerations related to preparticipation screening for cardiovascular abnormalities in competitive athletes. *Circulation* **115**: 1643–55

Maron, B.J., Thompson, P.D., Ackerman, M.J., et al. (2007). Recommendations and considerations related to pre-participation screening for cardiovascular abnormalities in competitive athletes: 2007 update: a scientific statement from the American Heart Association Council on Nutrition, Physical Activity, and Metabolism: endorsed by the American College of Cardiology Foundation *Circulation* **115**: 1643–55. (Consensus statement from the American Heart Association advocating use of a patient/family history and physical exam for the preparticipation evaluation, and reaffirming position against universal ECG screening in athletes.)

Wilson, M.G., Basavarajaiah, S., Whyte, G.P., et al. (2008). Efficacy of personal symptom and family history questionnaires when screening for inherited cardiac pathologies: the role of electrocardiography. *Br J Sports Med* **42**: 207–11.

General medical emergencies

:☼: Diabetes mellitus

While *hyper*glycaemia is rarely a pitch-side emergency, *hypo*glycaemia can cause brain damage or death, but fortunately is easily treatable.

Hypoglycaemia

Occurs when blood sugar is less than 3 mmol/L (but treat if less than 4 mmol/L and symptomatic).

Hypoglycaemia is usually caused by inadequate carbohydrate intake, excessive exercise, oral hypoglycaemic drugs or excessive insulin administration. It may also be the result of faulty glucose readings.

▶ Any athlete found unconscious should be assumed to be hypoglycaemic until proven otherwise. Likewise, any athlete who becomes aggressive and agitated should have hypoglycaemia excluded as a cause for their presentation.

Look for signs/symptoms such as:

- Sweating, anxiety, pallor, hunger tremor, *progressing to*
- Cold peripheries (driven by the sympathetic nervous system), tachycardia, headache, and dizziness, *progressing to*
- Confusion, behavioural change (such as aggressiveness and agitation), slurred speech, focal neurological deficit (due to neuroglucopaenia).

Ultimately, there will be loss of consciousness and possible seizure activity. Management depends on the conscious level of the athlete, with the aim to prevent progression from a mild episode to a severe one.

▶ Ask for help and do not leave the athlete alone.

- If alert and co-operative, repeat the blood glucose
- Provide a rapidly-acting carbohydrate, such as a concentrated sugar drink, sweet tea, and sweets or chocolate
- An alternative is to administer 30–50 g oral glucose gel, such as Glucogel® (40% dextrose gel). This may be more appealing to the athlete who is less co-operative and reluctant to drink
- Follow this up by administering a more sustained release of carbohydrate, such as bananas or sandwiches
- In athletes who are unconscious, assess and manage the airway, breathing, and circulation (A, B, Cs) as described in 📖 pp.13–14
- Medical management involves an IV injection of glucose and/or an intramuscular (IM) injection of glucagon. Glucose can be administered in varying concentrations. Aim to give 25 g by either 125 mL of 20%, 250 mL of 10%. Flush the cannula with saline, as concentrated dextrose is highly irritating to veins. Patients should regain consciousness or become coherent within a few minutes, although complete recovery may lag by up to an hour
- Repeat the blood glucose measurement and transfer to a place of safety, such as hospital, for readings to be repeated hourly until they become stable
- If the athlete has over-dosed on long-acting insulin or an oral hypoglycaemic drug, set up 500 mL 5–10% dextrose IV infusion to run over 5 h for transfer to hospital.

Note: There is no place for buccal glucose solutions in the unconscious or fitting patient:

- Some blood glucose readers may not be particularly accurate in assessing low blood sugars—if an athlete presents with symptoms, but a low end of normal BM then treat as for a mild hypo.
- If an athlete has a low sugar, but is asymptomatic, repeat the reading.
- If still low then assume asymptomatic hypoglycaemia and treat without waiting for symptoms to occur.
- Remember glycogen stores may be low especially in an athlete who has been exercising for a long period of time. In this situation, glucose is preferable to glucagon.

Considerations for the doctor

Review the athlete's current medication, inspecting all drugs taken.

- Consider other, much rarer causes of hypoglycaemia, including acute liver failure and acute alcohol consumption
- Recurrent hypoglycaemia may herald diabetic kidney disease. Poor kidney function reduces the need for insulin, which is partially metabolized by the kidney
- Betablockers mask the warning signs of hypoglycaemia
- Individuals with well-controlled diabetes are more at risk of hypoglycaemia and are less sensitive to developing signs/symptoms. These individuals develop neurological signs early with fewer warning signs
- Is there any possibility that the episode may have been self-inflicted?

Considerations for the insulin-dependent athlete

Different types of exercise in different environmental conditions can have variable effects on glucose. Advice should include:

- When exercising away from home, remember to carry carbohydrates that provide short-term energy, such as glucose drinks and fruit, as well as long-acting energy, such as nuts and wholemeal bread
- Carry out training when blood glucose is above fasting level, but not high. 1–2 h after a meal is ideal
- Develop the habit of measuring your blood glucose before, during (where practical) and after exercise. This gives a better understanding of personal carbohydrate and insulin requirements; which can be tailored to avoid detrimental fluctuations in blood glucose levels
- Athletes need approximately 15–30 g glucose for every 30 min of high intensity exercise
- Prolonged exercise (>2 h) usually necessitates regular carbohydrate consumption throughout to avoid hypoglycaemia
- Symptoms of dehydration can be mistaken for low blood sugars. Ensure you consume plenty of fluids before, during and after exercise
- Remember that after intensive exercise, your blood glucose may continue to drop for several hours
- Carbohydrate ingestion after exercise restocks your muscle stores and prevents low blood glucose
- Try not to drink alcohol after you exercise as it lowers blood glucose levels further and exacerbates dehydration.

Hyperglycaemia

Hyperglycaemia occurs in diabetics due to acute illness, steroids, and faulty testing. Hyperglycaemia in non-diabetics may be caused by glucose intolerance in the context of acute illness, such as infection or myocardial infarction; steroids, and faulty readings.

Do not over-react to mildly raised blood glucose (e.g. 12 mmol/L) on a single test. Diabetic ketoacidosis (DKA) or hyper-osmolar complications may take days to develop.

Diagnosis of DKA involves:
- Hyperglycaemia(usually >14 mmol/L) in association with
- Metabolic acidosis
- Ketones in blood and urine.

In the majority of cases, you will not have access to blood tests. Even if you have access to urine testing for ketones the athlete is usually so dehy-drated they will struggle to provide a sample of urine for testing.

Metabolic acidosis should be strongly suspected in a patient who has an ongoing high respiratory rate that cannot be attributed to any other cause as they try to blow off the acid that has built up. There may be a smell of ketones on the athletes breath—similar to nail polish (caused by acetone).

- Assess A, B, Cs and check the blood glucose
- Measure blood pressure (BP) and check for urinary ketones if possible
- Organize transfer to hospital for insulin sliding scale and to prevent progression to DKA if:
  - Blood glucose remains elevated and urinary ketones are positive
  - The blood glucose is >20 mmol/L
  - The athlete is hypotensive or unwell, e.g. drowsy, confused, gastrointestinal (GI) upset (abdominal pain, nausea, or vomiting)
- Set up 1000 mL IV saline for transfer to hospital. The rate of infusion should be adjusted according to level of dehydration and presence of cardiac disease.

▶ In managing DKA, the mainstay of treatment is fluid resuscitation— do not commence on IV or subcutaneous (SC) insulin pre-hospital.

Hyperglycaemia hyperosmolar state is a condition usually occurring in patients with Type 2 diabetes and is rarely seen in the young athlete who is far more likely to present with DKA. In this condition there is marked hyperglycaemia without acidosis or ketones. Treatment is again to correct the associated dehydration and does not involve insulin first line.

Considerations for the doctor

Non-insulin dependent diabetics may require insulin to maintain blood glucose control during episodes of acute illness.

Individuals with blood glucose >20 mmol/L are more at risk of DKA during intensive exercise. This is because the hormone response to exercise (glucagons, catecholamines, growth hormone, and glucocorticosteroids) is counter-regulatory to insulin at a time when there is already a lack of circulating insulin. This can rapidly increase blood glucose levels.

True laboratory glucose measurements are often higher and are more accurate than pitch-side capillary readings.

⬡ Acute exacerbations of asthma

There are athletes with asthma who train and compete within all sporting disciplines without significant impedance to their activities. Athletes who participate in outdoor sports are more likely to be exposed to common triggers, such as pollen and grass, although indoor arenas also harbour allergens, such as chalk dust or chlorine.

- The classic presentation is wheeze, breathlessness, and cough
- Exercise-induced asthma (EIA) due to airway mucosa irritation by dry and/or cold air is increasingly recognized in athletes
  - Presentation is with a combination of classic symptoms towards the end and after vigorous exercise
  - Typically these episodes resolve quickly and without concern
  - Acute asthma attacks are relatively common and usually resolve with inhalation of a short-acting beta-2 agonist
  - Rarely, an attack is severe and the athlete rapidly deteriorates; in this potentially life-threatening situation, prompt recognition and management is crucial.

It is always important to bear in the mind the differential diagnosis associated with the presentation of shortness of breath.

- Anaphylaxis
- Pneumothorax
- Pulmonary embolism
- Pulmonary oedema—especially associated with altitude
- Pneumonia.

These are all important to consider, especially the diagnosis of anaphylaxis which can be more common in patients who have asthma.

- A panic attack is not an acceptable diagnosis unless all other causes of shortness of breath have been carefully considered and excluded by careful history and examination.
- Clinical examination and peak expiratory flow (PEFR; either as a percentage of the patient's known best, or estimated from their height and age) are vital in classifying the severity of the attack, and thus allowing appropriate pre-hospital treatment and referral to hospital.

The aim is to classify the exacerbation into 1 of the 3 subgroups below as detailed by the British Thoracic/SIGN Guidelines of 2008.

Classification of acute asthma

Moderate exacerbation
- Increasing symptoms
- PEF between 50–75% of best or predicted
- No features of acute severe asthma.

Severe exacerbation
Any *one* of:
- PEF 33–50% of best or predicted
- Respiratory rate ≥ 25/min

- Heart rate ≥ 110/min
- Inability to complete sentences in one breath.

Life-threatening exacerbation

Any *one* of:

- PEF <33% or unable to carry out
- Silent chest with feeble respiratory effort
- Cyanosed
- Bradycardic or hypotensive
- Exhausted
- Decreased GCS (anything <15).

Other indicators, such as blood gases are clearly not appropriate in the pre-hospital setting but will detect rising CO_2 levels, which is a pre-terminal finding.

Oxygen saturations may be monitored with the use of a portable saturation probe. Anything less than 92% while breathing air is indicative of a life-threatening exacerbation.

Treatment of acute asthma

- Sit the athlete up to aid lung expansion and reassure
- Assess and classify the athlete into one of the 3 categories as above. Note that peak expiratory flow rate (PEFR) is vital
- Note past medical history; risk of severity increases with past history of hospital admission for asthma, ventilation, >3 types of asthma drugs, and repeated presentations to Emergency Department
- If PEFR is 75% or more, and there are no features of a moderate exacerbation then the management starts with inhaled bronchodilators (e.g. salbutamol, terbutaline) and reassess, including PEFR
- If there are any features of a moderate, severe, or life-threatening exacerbation, *then commence oxygen at as high a flow rate as possible— ideally 15 L/min* via non-rebreathable facemask (CO_2 retention is never an issue at this stage.)
- Commence nebulized beta-2-agonist, i.e. salbutamol 5 mg driven by oxygen, rather than air
- In severe asthma or asthma where there has been a poor response to the initial nebulizer consider continuous nebs and also add ipratropium bromide 0.5 mg to the beta-2-agonist
- In all cases of acute asthma give po prednisolone 50 mg for 5 days
- If there is no significant clinical response to bronchodilator therapy, or any of the following are present:
  - Unable to complete sentences in one breath
  - PEFR <50% of best or predicted
  - Respiratory rate >25 min
  - Heart rate >120 bpm *(NB. Beta-2-agonists may cause tachycardia)*
  - Hypotensive (systolic blood pressure (SBP) <100 mmHg)
  - Feeble breath sounds or 'silent chest'
  - Cyanosis or O_2 saturations <92%
  - Arrange urgent transfer to Emergency Department.
- Exhaustion, confusion, or coma may require intubation to assist breathing and maximize oxygenation. This should be only be attempted by those adequately trained and competent in a pre-hospital setting.
- Note that routine prescription of antibiotics is unnecessary.

☠ Anaphylaxis

Anaphylaxis is an immunological mediated systemic response resulting from the second exposure of a patient to an allergen with which they have already had previous sensitization (Fig. 8.1). It is a Type 1 immunoglobulin E (IgE) mediated response.

- An *anaphylactoid* reaction is clinically indistinguishable from anaphylaxis but is not the result of an immune mediated response
- Common allergens include nuts, strawberries, stings, and non-steroidal anti-inflammatories, such as diclofenac or ibuprofen.

An athlete may or may not have previously suffered from anaphylaxis, and thus may or may not be aware of the symptoms to look out for, or the treatments they require. Being aware as a team clinician that any of your athletes have allergies and the extent of these allergies is paramount in allowing you to consider the diagnosis and administer treatment.

Clinical manifestations

- *Airway:* swelling of tongue or mucosal surfaces, i.e. lips
- *Stridor:* hoarse voice
- *Breathing:* wheeze, increased respiratory rate
- *Circulation:* tachycardia, hypotension, increase capillary refill time
- *Skin:* flushed, itchy, urticaria
- *GI:* diarrhoea, vomiting.

Distinguishing between allergy and anaphylaxis

Anaphylaxis should be immediately suspected and treated if there is:

- Rapid progression of symptoms
- Skin or mucosal changes in association with either,
  - Airway compromise, *and/or*
  - Respiratory compromise, *and/or*
  - Circulatory compromise, i.e. decreased BP

That is, adrenaline IM is only required in the presence of a compromise of A, B, or C.

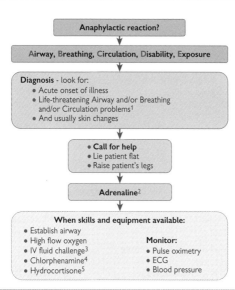

Anaphylactic reaction?

↓

Airway, Breathing, Circulation, Disability, Exposure

↓

Diagnosis - look for:
- Acute onset of illness
- Life-threatening Airway and/or Breathing and/or Circulation problems[1]
- And usually skin changes

↓

- **Call for help**
- Lie patient flat
- Raise patient's legs

↓

Adrenaline[2]

↓

When skills and equipment available:
- Establish airway
- High flow oxygen
- IV fluid challenge[3]
- Chlorphenamine[4]
- Hydrocortisone[5]

Monitor:
- Pulse oximetry
- ECG
- Blood pressure

[1] **Life-threatening problems:**
Airway: swelling, hoarseness, stridor
Breathing: rapid breathing, wheeze, fatigue, cyanosis, SpO_2 <92%, confusion
Circulation: pale, clammy, low blood pressure, faintness, drowsy/coma

[2] **Adrenaline** *(give IM unless experienced with IV adrenaline)*
IM doses of 1:1000 adrenaline (repeat after 5 min if no better)
- Adult   500 micrograms IM (0.5 mL)
- Child more than 12 years: 500 micrograms IM (0.5 mL)
- Child 6–12 years: 300 micrograms IM (0.3 mL)
- Child less than 6 years: 150 micrograms IM (0.15 mL)

Adrenaline IV to be given **only by experienced specialists**
Titrate: Adults 50 micrograms; Children 1 microgram/kg

[3] **IV fluid challenge:**
Adult - 500–1000 mL
Child - crystalloid 20 mL/kg

Stop IV colloid
if this might be the cause
of anaphylaxis

	[4] Chlorphenamine (IM or slow IV)	[5] Hydrocortisone (IM or slow IV)
Adult or child more than 12 years	10 mg	200 mg
Child 6–12 years	5 mg	100 mg
Child 6 months to 6 years	2.5 mg	50 mg
Child less than 6 months	250 micrograms/kg	25 mg

Fig. 8.1 Anaphylaxis algorithm. Reproduced with the kind permission of the Resuscitation Council (UK).

☢ Seizures

(See 📖 also p.38)
Focus of management of epilepsy or seizures of any aetiology is clearly prevention. When a seizure occurs, the management is prescriptive. Being prepared is vital—ensure you have access to the correct equipment including a mobile phone.

- Status epilepticus is defined as seizure activity ongoing for more than 30 min, or repeated seizures without consciousness being regained
- It is a life-threatening condition with a high mortality, the rate of which increases with the increasing duration of the seizure.

Management aims

- Maintain an airway
- Terminate the seizure if not self-terminated within 2 min
- Identify potential reversible causes namely *hypoglycaemia*.

⚠ Remember that cardiac arrest caused by ventricular fibrillation may present as a short-lived seizure. Check for a pulse in all patients suffering from a seizure.

When to phone an ambulance

- Status epilepticus
- Seizure lasting longer than 5 min
- Athletes first seizure
- Seizure as a result of injury
- Injury resulting from seizure
- Multiple seizures.

Medications

There are a number of medications belonging to the benzodiazepine family that can be used to terminate seizures.

All members of the benzodiazepine family have a similar side-effect profile, such as respiratory depression and hypotension. The extent of these effects varies between drugs, but being familiar with these effects is paramount, as is having the correct equipment to deal with them.

Management of seizures

- Maintain airway. Use a naso- or oropharyngeal airway if tolerated. (The latter may be impossible to insert due to teeth clenching)
- Administer 15 L of oxygen as available
- Check for a pulse
- If fitting for more than 2 min:
  - Obtain IV access and check a blood glucose monitor (BM)
  - Administer either lorazepam 4 mg IV or diazepam 10 mg IV (buccal or intranasal route of benzodiazepine administration may be more appropriate)
- Phone an ambulance if fitting for more than 5 min

- If still fitting after 10 min
  - Administer second dose of benzodiazepine
  - *Ensure ambulance has been called.*

:✪: **Acute onset shortness of breath**

The presenting complaint of shortness of breath (SOB) raises the potential of many differential diagnoses. The ability to distinguish between these causes is usually based on a sound clinical history and examination findings, with very little routinely required in terms of immediate investigations. PEFR and oxygen saturations are the exceptions, and can be very helpful pitchside.

- Asthma (see 📖 p.94)
- Anaphylaxis (see 📖 p.96)
- Simple pneumothorax (see 📖 p. 169)
- Tension pneumothorax (see 📖 p. 170)
- Pulmonary embolism (PTE)
- Pulmonary oedema
- Pneumonia
- Metabolic acidosis.

Pulmonary embolism

Very unusual presentation to a team clinician but may be seen as a result of a deep venous thrombosis (DVT) that migrates from the lower leg to the lungs. May present suddenly as a cardiac arrest or over the course of a few weeks with episodes of SOB, with or without chest pain that appear to settle spontaneously.

- Look for evidence of a DVT with a history directed at assessing risk factors such as previous DVT, lower limb immobilization in cast, recent flight
- Examination should look for calf swelling and tenderness
- The chest will usually yield little in terms of examination, with normal lung fields a common finding
- Saturations will typically be low and may be difficult to pick up if the patient is shocked
- Administer high flow oxygen as soon as possible
- Obtain IV access and commence fluids if shocked
- Immediately transfer to hospital for ongoing management and investigations.

Pulmonary oedema

The most likely presentation to the team physician will be of either pulmonary oedema induced at altitude (see 📖 p.72) or as an acute episode of left ventricular failure in the case of a more elderly patient.

If clinically suspected by history such as previous episodes, onset when lying flat, associated chest pain, or by examination, such as tachycardia, bilateral crepitations, patient cold, and clammy, lower leg oedema, then apply high flow oxygen, obtain IV access and administer furosemide. Nitrates are likely to be required and can be given as long as systolic BP is maintained above 90 mmHg.

Pneumonia

Unusual to present hyper-acutely with sudden shortness of breath, and more common to present with a progression of symptoms including SOB in association with cough (which usually becomes productive in the case of bacterial pneumonias), pyrexia, general malaise, anorexia, pleuritic chest pain, rigors.

- Examination may reveal crepitations, tachypnoea, tachycardia, and decreased saturations
- Hospital referral will be required in anyone who is hypotensive, saturations <94%, significant co-morbidity or deterioration despite treatment with oral fluids, anti-pyretics, such as paracetamol, and antibiotics in the case of clinical bacterial pneumonia
- Antibiotics should be prescribed according to local policy, i.e. amoxicillin as first line primary care treatment.

Metabolic acidosis

It is worth remembering that someone who becomes progressively SOB may not actually be suffering from a primary respiratory problem and instead may be suffering from a buildup of acid.

- The acidosis is best cleared from the body by blowing off carbon dioxide via the lungs—resulting in an increase in the respiratory rate
- In the young the most common cause of metabolic acidosis is DKA (see 🔲 p.92) or renal failure resulting in uraemia
- Pointers to the diagnosis may be from the history—especially in diabetics with a ketotic odour
- Patients will usually have a clinically clear chest and are likely to saturate at 99–100% unless peripherally shut down
- Note that in the case of a PTE, where the chest may again also be clear, the saturations are almost certainly highly likely to be abnormal
- Other causes of metabolic acidosis include toxins such as aspirin, and the potential of an overdose (accidental or deliberate) should also be considered
- Treatment is directed to reversing the cause of the acidosis though this should begin by maximizing oxygen uptake with high flow oxygen and fluid resuscitation good first line measures especially when the diagnosis is in doubt
- Transfer to hospital will always be required in these patients.

☼: Chest pain emergencies

There are many potential causes of chest pain from problems that affect the skin (such as shingles) through the musculoskeletal system (such as muscular tear, costochondritis, fractured ribs) and finishing with the vital organs—lungs (including pleura) heart, and mediastinum.

- Pain may also radiate from other structures such as those of the upper abdomen, notably the stomach
- A thorough history and examination should allow the causes of chest pain to be narrowed down, and hopefully a firm diagnosis made.

▶▶ If you are unclear of the cause of chest pain then assume it to be significant, and seek assistance and transfer to hospital.

Many of the potentially life-threatening causes of chest pain have been discussed elsewhere in the book most notably in the pre-ceding pages of this chapter.

The pre-hospital key to diagnosis lies firmly in the history and to a lesser extent on examination. A structured approach to assessment should always be thoroughly carried out and regardless of the aetiology of the pain. A similar pre-hospital treatment plan can be commenced.

Pain can be categorized in many ways, but one of the easiest involves dividing into either pleuritic or non-pleuritic, where pleuritic pain is classically sharp in nature and worsened by breathing.

This is not set in stone, i.e. pericarditis may not be pleuritic in nature but it is worth considering the different causes in this manner to be clear in your mind what you are assessing for.

Potential pleuritic causes of chest pain

- Pneumothorax (📖 pp.169–71)
- Pulmonary Embolism
- Pneumonia
- Pericarditis (+/– Myocarditis)
- Musculoskeletal.

Pericarditis

- Inflammation or infection of the pericardium can result in fluid accumulating in the pericardial sac. At a critical volume, this fluid prevents the heart from contracting resulting in cardiogenic shock. The volume necessary to cause tamponade will vary depending on the length of time it takes to accumulate
- Pericarditis typically causes a sharp pain that may worsen with movement and potentially with breathing. The pain is classically worsened when lying flat and eased when sitting forward
- Pericarditis may result from viral infections, but tuberculosis (TB) should also be considered especially in anyone presenting with a secondary pericardial effusion
- Assessment may reveal very little though a pericardial rub should be looked for at the left lower sternal edge. Muffled heart sounds, raised jugular venous pressure (JVP) and hypotension (Beck's triad) would suggest cardiac tamponade necessitating immediate transfer to hospital

- Management of anyone with pericarditis involves maximizing oxygenation with high flow oxygen and supplying analgesia. Assessment in hospital should be carried out to allow an ECG to be undertaken to confirm the diagnosis and an echocardiogram (ECHO) performed to exclude an effusion.

Musculoskeletal

- Note that musculoskeletal causes of pain, whilst very common are diagnoses of exclusion made after every other cause has been considered
- In the case of trauma, anyone in whom you truly suspect fractured ribs should be closely monitored and consideration made to refer for X-ray—not to diagnose the rib fracture, but to exclude concomitant underlying lung pathology, such as pneumothorax
- Pre-hospital management, common to all of the above conditions involves commencing high flow oxygen and analgesia to the patient
- Specific treatments may need to be administered, such as decompressing a tension pneumothorax or administering antibiotics
- Entonox® is not an appropriate analgesic agent in these cases, as oxygenation should be maximized.

▶▶ Anyone with abnormal observations and pleuritic chest pain will require referral to hospital.

Non–pleuritic causes of chest pain

- Myocardial infarction (MI) or acute coronary syndrome (ACS)
- Aortic Dissection
- Pancreatitis
- Gastritis.

Myocardial infarction/acute coronary syndrome

This is an unusual presentation for a young athlete, although certain drugs (such as anabolic steroids and cocaine) can predispose the patient to suffering from an MI/ACS. It will more commonly present in the older athlete who may or may not have risk factors for ischaemic heart disease, such as smoking, hypertension, or a past history of angina.

- Pain is classically described as tightness, heaviness, crushing pain that may radiate to either arm or the neck.
- There may be associated shortness of breath, sweating, or nausea.
- Pain that lasts for longer than 15 min and is of this nature should be assumed to be a result of an MI/ACS and an ambulance phoned for the patient.
- The distinction between an MI/ACS is not important in the pre-hospital setting as treatment with oxygen, aspirin, sublingual nitrate, and IV opiate if available is the basis for treating both conditions.

Aortic dissection

Again, an unusual presentation (incidence not clear as failure to initially diagnose the condition occurs in up to a third of cases), although commoner in some sports, such as basketball in which there is a higher incidence of athletes with Marfans syndrome.

- This condition along with others such as Ehlers–Danlos, syphilis, and hypertension predisposes the aorta to a weakness in the medial layer of the vessel
- It is this weakness that results in a tear in the intima and resulting dissection of the aorta
- Pain will depend on which aspect of the aorta is affected and it may change in position as the tear evolves
- Anterior chest pain may be found in ascending or aortic root dissections, with neck pain in arch dissection
- Pain from the descending aorta is classically described as tearing interscapular pain.

▶ Pain usually *maximal at onset*, which may help to distinguish from MI/ACS.

- Examination should assess for pulse including both radial arteries.
- Assess BP in both arms although it should be remembered that it can be normal to have differences of up to 20 mmHg between arms.
- BP maybe high or low, with hypotension a poor prognostic indicator.
- Listen to heart sounds for murmurs or muffled sounds that might suggest an associated effusion or tamponade.
- Listen to the chest for evidence of an effusion.
- Pre-hospital treatment involves oxygenating and supplying analgesia with immediate transfer of the patient to the nearest hospital.

:Ö: Emergency causes of headache

- Headache is a common symptom that may occur as the result of many different pathologies both benign as well as life-threatening
- Most people will experience a headache significant enough to require analgesia at some point in their lives
- It is a common complaint and the key to identifying the life-threatening causes usually lies with taking an adequate history
- Best thought of as divided into traumatic and non-traumatic causes.

Traumatic causes

- Subdural haematoma (🕮 p.125)
- Extradural haematoma (🕮 p.125)
- Concussion (🕮 p. 122).

The history in these cases is usually evident with respect to trauma. The lucid interval prior to deterioration in conscious level is still an unfortunate classic presentation of an extra-dural and is the reason that serial neuro-observation should be routinely performed after every head injury and for a period not less than 24 h.

Non-traumatic causes

- Subarachnoid haemorrhage
- Meningitis/encephalitis
- Hypertensive crisis
- Temporal arteritis.

Certain 'red flags' in the history may help to point towards the cause of a life-threatening headache.

- Sudden onset—highly suggestive of subarachnoid headache (SAH)
- Most severe headache ever (SAH)
- Described as 'like being hit on the back of the head with a baseball bat' (SAH)
- Associated with a syncopal episode (SAH)
- Sudden onset of severe upper neck pain without palpable tenderness and good range of movement (SAH)
- Photophobia (SAH or meningitis)
- Neck stiffness (meningitis)
- Purpuric rash (meningitis)
- Associated fever (meningitis)
- Temporal headache (consider temporal arteritis especially if over 40 years old).

Subarachnoid haemorrhage

- Usually the result of rupture of a berry aneurysm or arteriovenous (AV) malformation
- Incidence varies between countries but is about 10:100,000/year
- Anyone who volunteers the information of pain like 'being hit on the back of the head' should be assumed to have a SAH until proven otherwise
- Involves admission to hospital for CT scan +/– lumbar puncture

- There may be vomiting in association with the occipital headache
- Mortality approaches 50%
- Key to treatment is identification and emergent referral to hospital.

Meningitis/encephalitis
- May be viral or bacterial
- May occur in isolation or together therefore treatment usually involves antibiotics and antivirals IV
- Symptoms may be rapid in onset (i.e. <24 h) in about 25% with the potential for a rapid deterioration in condition unless treated with antibiotics quickly
- Symptoms may be fairly non-specific, making diagnosis difficult
- Pyrexia, headache, vomiting, photophobia, and neck stiffness are classic textbook signs that may also be found in a number of other conditions making diagnosis difficult in times of influenza outbreak for example:
  - Bacterial meningitis can be caused by many different organisms including *Neisseria meningitidis* and *Strep pneumonia*. Pneumococcal meningitis has the highest incidence of mortality
  - Pre-hospital management involves pain relief, antiemetic, anti-pyretics, IM benzylpenicllin, and IV fluids if necessary.

Hypertensive crisis
It is common for BP to rise in response to pain. As such, an elevated BP may be a normal physiological finding in a patient suffering from headaches caused by migraines, for example:
- In contrast, someone who is suffering from a headache brought about by uncontrolled BP must be identified and treated in the hospital setting
- Usually in this setting the systolic BP will be >220 mmHg
- Refer immediately to hospital anyone who has symptomatic high BP.

Temporal arteritis
- Unusual under the age of 40 years
- Affects females more than males
- Important as a cause of headache associated with irreversible blindness
- Headache may be sudden and located to the temporal area
- Pain may be felt when combing the hair
- Hospital referral is necessary for erythrocyte sedimentation rate (ESR) and biopsy though treatment may commence with steroids in suspected cases without blood or biopsy test results.

☼ Palpitations

- Palpitations are a relatively common complaint. They are described as an awareness of a forceful and usually fast heart beat
- There are many causes of palpitations but the aim is distinguishing the benign ('skipped beat') from the life-threatening tachyarrythmias
- Palpitations may occur as an isolated symptom or may be associated with symptoms of syncope, chest pain, shortness of breath, or dizziness
- Any association with syncope mandates an immediate hospital assessment
- Chest pain will also usually result in a hospital admission though this may be avoided in an athlete who is known to suffer recurrent supraventrular tachycardias (SVT) and whose symptoms terminate with cessation of the SVT
- It is important to try to distinguish the rate and rhythm of the palpitations, the regularity of their onset as well as any precipitating or relieving factors
- History and examination are key.

History

- Is this an awareness of a 'skipped' beat, multiple beats, or a sustained episode of the heart racing?
- If racing then for how long?
- Are there any associated symptoms as described above?
- How often has this happened before?
- Is there anything you can do to make them stop?
- Have you had any previous cardiac history?
- Are you on any medications?
- Is there any family history of cardiac disease or sudden death?
- Is there a history of alcohol or cocaine abuse?

Remember iatrogenic causes of arrhythmias, such as over doseage of local anaesthetic.

Examination

This is based around the ABC principles described in 📖 Chapter 2.
 Check the pulse for evidence of a tachycardia with a rate above 100 bpm.

- Is it regular or irregular?
- What is the volume of the pulse?
- The blood pressure?
- Is the patient shocked or clinically well?

Investigation

- The ability to obtain a 12-lead ECG or even a rhythm strip should confirm the clincal findings with respect to the actual heart rate if caught in time
- It will also allow you to classify the tachycardia as either an SVT or VT
- Maximal heart rate is usually considered to be around 220 bpm minus age and it is highly unlikely that a sinus tachycardia would present at a rate greater than this.

Management of palpitations
See Fig. 8.2.
- Management is based on identifying the underlying driver for the tachycardia as either SVT or VT and treating the patient on the basis of their cardiovascular status
- A controlled pulse with occasional ectopic beats can usually be managed with simple reasssurance
- If you do not have access to an ECG then vagal manouevres may be performed on a stable patient with a tachycardia
- This will have no effect on VT, but may cardiovert an SVT
- Remember to check for a carotid bruit prior to performing carotid massage
- Any athlete suffering from palpitations will require a full cardiology work up including ECG and ECHO
- Blood tests may also be useful in identifying any electrolyte abnormalities, such as hypomagnesia, which may predispose to recurrent arrythmias.

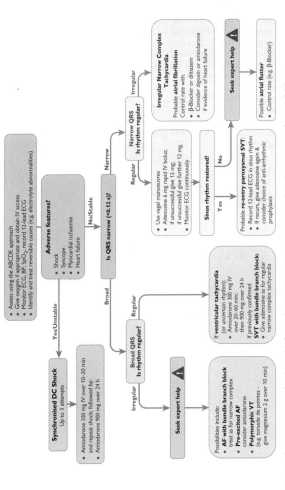

Fig. 8.2 Algorithm for management of tachycardia. Reproduced with the kind permission of the Resuscitation Council (UK).

Further reading

British Thoracic Guidelines/Scottish Intercollegiate Guidelines Network (2008, revised 2011). Available at: ℺ www.sign.ac.uk/pdf/qrg101.pdf.

Resuscitation Council. Available at: ℺ www.resus.org.uk.

Head injuries

Background

Head injury is common in contact sports ranging from minor injury with no neurological deficit through varying degrees of concussion to traumatic brain injury. The pitchside practitioner must be competent in assessment and management of head injuries with awareness of sequelae.

- In a recent National Confidential Enquiry into Patient Outcome and Death (NCEPOD) report 'Trauma: who cares' it was noted that in the UK, traumatic brain injury accounts for 15–20% of deaths between the ages of 5 and 35 years, with an incidence of 9 per 100,000 per year
- Outcome after head injury depends upon the initial severity of injury and also the extent of any subsequent complications and how these are managed
- Most of the patients who attend hospital after a head injury do not develop life-threatening or disabling complications in the acute stage. However, in a small, but important group of patients, outcome is made worse by a failure to either detect promptly or to deal adequately with complications
- There is a growing body of evidence that secondary insults occur frequently and exert a profound, adverse effect on out-come from severe head injury. It is therefore recommended that hypotension (systolic blood pressure (SBP) <90 mmHg) and hypoxia (PaO_2 <8 kPa) must be scrupulously avoided or treated immediately to avoid worsening outcome.

Pitchside equipment and pre-event preparation

Equipment
- Oxygen with reservoir bag mask
- Suction apparatus
- Airway adjuncts
- Full length spinal board with body and head straps
- Adjustable size cervical collar.

Pre-event preparation
- Contact local hospital to inform of event, ensure hospital has computed tomography (CT) scanning facilities available. Identify your nearest neurosurgical unit
- Assess ambulance provision at the event. Are paramedics needed? Is the team proficient in the log roll technique. Are they aware of their roles and responsibilities with a designated lead?
- Try to practice scenarios pre-event with medical and pitchside team
- Be aware of and make adjustments according to environmental conditions
- Ensure efficient access from pitch to medical room/ambulance for injured player
- Ensure all staff are aware of location of equipment and evacuation procedures.

☼ Pitchside assessment of head injury

- The pitchside practitioner must watch the sporting event in order to witness the mechanism of any injury, in a head injury particular attention is paid to any loss of consciousness
- Should the practitioner need to enter the field of play, they must ensure a safe approach
- This will usually involve ensuring that the match officials have stopped the play or event
- It is useful to have introduce yourself prior to the event and ensure that an agreement is reached as to how this will occur
- The approach to the patient will be the same as for any injured player (see 📖 Chapter 2).
  - **A:** airway
  - **B:** breathing
  - **C:** circulation
  - **D:** disability (assessed using the Glasgow Coma Scale or the AVPU) measure of response
  - **E:** exposure/environment.

AVPU scale

- A: Alert
- V: Responsive to Vocal stimuli only
- P: Responsive to Pain stimuli only
- U: Unresponsive.

Glasgow Coma Scale

Eye opening
- 4 Spontaneous
- 3 Verbal commands
- 2 Pain
- 1 None.

Best motor response
- 6 Obeys
- 5 Localizes
- 4 Withdraws
- 3 Abnormal flexion posturing
- 2 Abnormal extension posturing
- 1 None.

Best verbal response
- 5 Orientated
- 4 Disorientated or confused
- 3 Inappropriate words
- 2 Incomprehensible sounds
- 1 None

Potential cervical spine injuries

If loss of consciousness, assume C-spine injury:
- ABCDE + oxygen (12–15 L of 100% with reservoir bag) + C-spine immobilization. This can be carried out manually in the first instance. During transfer, 'triple immobilization' should be carried out, with a correctly sized rigid neck collar, sandbags (or equivalent) to either side of the head, and tape placed over the forehead and sandbags and attached to the extraction device, and the same replicated over the chin
- If evidence of airway obstruction, jaw thrust manoeuvre should be performed and/or an airway adjunct inserted after being correctly sized
- The patient should be log-rolled onto an extraction device, e.g. a long board or 'scoop' stretcher
- If the patient vomits then a log roll manoeuvre will be required to turn them onto their side.

If there is no loss of consciousness:
- Assessment of head injury and C-spine can be performed. Following injury player should be held in manual in line stabilization in supine position whilst assessment is carried out
- Practitioner must assess for any sign of gross neurological deficit including visual disturbance
- Player must be fully conscious, alert, and orientated in order to clear the C-spine:
  - Ask regarding neck pain and palpate cervical spine for tenderness or step deformity
  - Assess limb movement and ask regarding any paraesthesia or anaesthesia
  - Gently allow mobilization of the neck stopping and instituting immobilization if there is any pain and or resistance.

The Nexus guidelines (see Box 9.1) provide a validated guideline for the clearance of cervical spine injury (for further information see 📖 p.158).

Box 9.1 The NEXUS clinical criteria for c-spine clearance

1. The absence of tenderness at the posterior midline of the cervical spine
2. The absence of a focal neurological deficit
3. A normal level of alertness
4. No evidence of intoxication
5. Absence of clinically apparent pain that might distract the patient from the pain of a cervical spine injury

⊙ Minor head injury management

For the purposes of this chapter a minor head injury is classified as one which had neither loss of consciousness nor neurological deficit evident. Principals of management are the same as all head injuries with a primary survey—ABCDE in the first instance. This is followed by clearance of the C-spine, assessment of neurological function, Modified Maddock's questions (Box 9.2), and gradual return to upright position and then fluid replacement.

- Answering any question incorrectly is suggestive of concussion and mandates removal from the pitch
- Whether the athlete stays on the pitch or is removed, continual reassessment is recommended. If the player continues the practitioner must watch their movements closely and ask regarding symptoms at breaks in play and at half-time and full-time
- If it is decided to remove from play a decision needs to be made regarding transfer to hospital. Should there be any neurological deficit or C-spine injury suspicion then player must be sent for further investigation and management
- If player is deemed unable to continue yet no suspicion of traumatic brain injury then player must be monitored by practitioner for at least the first hour post injury and then followed up with head injury advice
- Beware distracting injuries such as scalp laceration and ensure you fully access the potential head and neck injury first. Ensure all wounds are fully cleaned and explored prior to closure.
  - Reassess at end of game with full neurological examination and Maddock's questions.
  - Ensure the player is monitored for at least the 1st hour post-injury.
  - When the patient is discharged from your care they must have a responsible adult to monitor them for the next 24 h.
  - Information should be provided to the patient and carer, and backed up with written advice for them to follow (Box 9.3). This should include information on treatment of a minor head injury
- It is imperative to keep thorough medical notes of the injury and management
- It is useful to have head injury advice sheets readily available to give to the player having explained the process with their responsible adult who will be with them for the next 24 h
- These should contain contact details of club medical staff to ensure any deterioration is reported and appropriate management instigated
- The head injury advice sheet should also contain information about symptoms the player may experience (see Box 9.4). The development of any of these symptoms mandates urgent medical reassessment.

Box 9.2 Modified Maddock's questions

1. At what venue are we?
2. Which half is it?
3. Who scored last?
4. What team did we play last week?
5. Did we win the last game?

Box 9.3 Home with head injury advice

- 'Brain rest'
- No alcohol
- Minimize stimulants, e.g. TV, computer
- Ensure patient is not alone over first 24 hr
- Do not drive
- Ensure adequate hydration

Box 9.4 Signs of significant head injury

Include:
- Progressively worsening headache
- Repeated vomiting
- Visual disturbance
- Excessive drowsiness, irritability or altered personality
- Dizziness, loss of balance, or convulsions
- Blood or clear fluid, leaking from the nose or ear
- New deafness in one or both ears
- Unusual breathing patterns
- Loss of use of part of the body
- Confusion, strange behaviour, any problems understanding or speaking

☼ Significant head injury management

A significant head injury is classified for the purposes of this chapter, as injury causing witnessed loss of consciousness and/or neurological deficit on examination (see Box 9.4 for signs of significant head injury).

Management, as with all head injuries, begins with the primary survey:
- ABCDE + oxygen (12–15 L 100% with a reservoir bag)
- C-spine immobilization should be instigated if there is loss of consciousness as practitioner cannot clear a C-spine in an unconscious player
- In an unconscious player's airway compromise may require a jaw thrust, as well as airway adjuncts
- If the player suffers a seizure it is important to maintain in line immobilization as much as possible, however, with violent movements this will need to be gentle support, rather than rigid immobilization. Likewise oxygen therapy should be continued even in violent movements by placing mask in close vicinity to airway
- If possible full neurological assessment should be instigated. Signs and symptoms requiring hospital transfer for CT to exclude cerebral pathology include:
  - Depressed GCS below 14, which continues after initial presentation
  - Focal neurological signs
  - Suspicion of skull fracture, open or depressed
  - Signs of fracture at base of skull (haemotympanum, 'panda' eyes, cerebrospinal fluid leakage from ears or nose, Battle's sign)
  - Significant progressive headache, excessive drowsiness, visual disturbance, repeated vomiting
  - Post-traumatic seizure
  - Amnesia of events more than 30 min prior to injury.

It is recommended to call ahead with status update of injured player to hospital. Having established links pre event the hospital will be aware of event and possibility of injuries being brought in.

It is imperative to once again ensure thorough documentation of the injury and subsequent management, it is also important to communicate clearly with the player if applicable and with paramedics, ambulance staff, and the member of your medical team who may accompany player to hospital if transfer is to occur.

⚠ Concussion management

At the International Conference on Concussion in sport, held in Zurich in 2008, a consensus statement was produced that defined concussion as: 'a complex pathophysiological process affecting the brain, induced by traumatic biomechanical forces. Several common features that incorporate clinical, pathological, and biomechanical injury constructs that may be utilized in defining the nature of a concussive head injury include:

- Concussion may be caused either by a direct blow to the head, face, neck, or elsewhere on the body with an 'impulsive' force transmitted to the head
- Concussion typically results in the rapid onset of short-lived impairment of neurological function that resolves spontaneously
- Concussion may result in neuropathological changes, but the acute clinical symptoms largely reflect a functional disturbance, rather than a structural injury
- Concussion results in a graded set of clinical symptoms that may or may not involve loss of consciousness. Resolution of the clinical and cognitive symptoms typically follows a sequential course; however, it is important to note that in a small percentage of cases, post-concussive symptoms may be prolonged
- No abnormality on standard structural neurological imaging studies is seen in concussion.

The suspected diagnosis of concussion can include one or more of the following clinical domains:

- *Symptoms:* somatic (e.g. headache), cognitive (e.g. feeling like in a fog) and/or emotional symptoms (e.g. lability).
- *Physical signs:* e.g. loss of consciousness, amnesia
- *Behavioural changes:* e.g. irritability
- *Cognitive impairment:* e.g. slowed reaction times
- *Sleep disturbance:* e.g. drowsiness.'

The complexity of the definition demonstrates the complexity of the condition.

- ⚠ It is important to appreciate that consciousness may still be retained and that imaging studies will be normal
- During pitchside assessment of head injury brief neuropsychological tests that assess attention and memory function have been shown to be practical and effective to diagnose concussion. Such tests include the Maddock's questions
- Concussion may be immediately apparent and necessitate removal from play or it may present post-event with the player having continued to play on. It is important to repeat the Maddock's questions as part of the practitioner's full neurological assessment following head injury if a player has continued
- If concussion is diagnosed this will mandate a graded return to play to allow symptom resolution. Further tools to assess concussion include the Sport Concussion Assessment Tool (SCAT)

- Baseline neuropsychological testing (e.g. Impact, Cog Sport) can aid as an indicator of return to play, allowing comparison of cognitive function against the players own healthy baseline
- Symptom resolution is, however, the key to return to play
- △ The cornerstone of concussion management is physical and cognitive rest until symptoms resolve and then a graded programme of exertion prior to medical clearance and return to play
- Typical resolution of symptoms is achieved in 7–10 days in 80–90% of cases. In some sports there are guidelines and minimum time restrictions set for return to player, e.g. RFU 21 days depending on medical supervision
- Graded return to activity is in various stages with at least 24 h between each stage, if symptoms recur at any stage then the protocol dictates dropping back to the last asymptomatic stage and then progressing once more. An important consideration in return to play is that concussed athletes should not only be symptom-free but also should not be taking any pharmacological agents/medications that may mask or modify the symptoms of concussion
- A detailed concussion history taken at baseline while the player is healthy provides important information in the event of a concussion. It is important to ascertain the severity of impact/injury, return to play time (Box 9.5), and frequency of concussive episodes
- There is little evidence to suggest that repetitive head injuries result in 'second impact syndrome' (rapid, severe cerebral oedema following head injury sustained, whilst still symptomatic from previous concussion) or cumulative damage. Indeed, it seems more likely that there is a genetic predisposition to concussion incidence and/or outcome (i.e. some athletes may be more prone to concussion and take longer to recover from them)
- Where an athlete has a history of previous concussions medical staff may proceed with extra caution when making return to play decisions.

Box 9.5 Graduated return to play (RTP) protocol

- Rehabilitation stage
- Functional exercise at each stage of rehabilitation
- Objective of each stage

Stage 1
- No activity
- Complete physical and cognitive rest
- Recovery

Stage 2
- Light aerobic exercise
- Walking, swimming, or stationary cycling, keeping intensity at 70% maximum predicted heart rate. No resistance training
- Increase heart rate

Stage 3
- Sport-specific exercise
- Sport specific drills. No head impact activities
- Add movement

Stage 4
- Non-contact training drills
- Progression to more complex training drills. May start progressive resistance training
- Exercise, co-ordination, and cognitive load

Stage 5
- Full contact practice
- Following medical clearance participate in normal training activities
- Restore confidence and assess functional skills by coaching staff

Stage 6
- Return to play
- Normal game play

✪: Subdural haematoma

The traumatic injury causes blood to be released into the subdural space. This is classically due to rupture of the bridging cerebral veins.

- There is usually a brief loss of consciousness and period of confusion. It is more common in the older athlete
- As the mass increases further symptoms will develop. These will depend on the location of the haematoma, but can be quite subtle with increasing headache or vomiting, being the only early symptoms
- The injury may be associated with a substantial soft tissue injury to the head and possible associated cranial vault fracture, but these do not have to be present
- Late features of intracranial pressure increase from the mass may include ipsilateral third nerve palsy
- Prognosis from an acute subdural event will often depend more on damage to the cerebral parenchyma from the force of injury, rather than the presence of a subdural bleed itself.

✪: Extradural haematomas

This results from a direct blow to the skull. This causes deformation of the skull and tearing of the vessels associated with the extradura. It is commonly associated with fractures in adults, but is also seen in children due to the flexibility of the skull.

- 50% of the bleeding is associated with the middle meningeal artery
- 33% are associated with venous bleeds
- Fractures of the skull can also lead to mass effect from accumulating blood
- The patient will usually present with an injury associated with loss of consciousness
- The patient may then appear to return to normal
- However after a variable period of time, symptoms of raised intracranial pressure will start usually with headaches or vomiting
- Sometimes the presentation can be dramatic with a patient proceeding from apparent normal consciousness to deeply unconscious in a matter of minutes
- Prompt surgical evacuation is required for all expanding extradural haematomas.

✪: Diffuse cerebral swelling

- This can occur after only minor head injuries and children appear to be particularly at risk
- There is rapid cerebral swelling leading to a rise in the intracranial pressure. The mechanism for this is not well understood
- Treatment is the same for all types of brain injury with an ABCDE approach.

☼ Intracerebral haematomas

- These can occur in response to a direct blow or from movement of the brain within the skull vault (leading to the coup and conta-coup injury patterns)
- Signs and symptoms will depend on the location of the injury within the brain parenchyma.

① Scalp injuries

The scalp is made up of five distinct layers
- **S**: skin
- **C**: connective tissue
- **A**: aponeurosis
- **L**: loose areolar tissue
- **P:** periosteum

The scalp has an excellent blood supply and can allow an extra-cranial haematoma to expand readily. Patients can lose a large amount of blood through a scalp wound leading to hypotension, which is a poor prognostic sign for an intracranial injury.

Remember, however, to exclude other causes of blood loss, which you should assess for as part of the circulation assessment. Treatment to prevent blood loss will initially consist of direct pressure. Suturing will also help to control haemorrhage. This usually requires a large curved needle.

The evaluation of a scalp wound should include palpation for a possible depressed fracture, identification, and removal of foreign bodies and careful cleaning with copious amounts of water.

When closing the wound the aponeurosis must be closed with interrupted sutures and then the skin closed over it. However, in an emergency all layers can be closed together. For minor injuries to the scalp, glue can be a quick and effective alternative.

During a sporting event, sutures are often placed quickly to prevent blood loss and to return the player to the field of play as soon as possible. On these occasions it is appropriate to remove the sutures after completion of the sport and to ensure thorough wound exploration and cleaning prior to repeating the suture of the wound for best cosmetic effect.

Further reading

Advanced Resuscitation and Emergency Aid course (2009). Available at: ℘ www.remosports. com/area-courses.

National Institute for Health and Clinical Excellence (NICE) (2007). *Head Injury Guide*. NICE, London.

(2008). Consensus Statement on Concussion in Sport. 3rd International Conference on Concussion in Sport, Zurich, November.

England Hockey: Concussion Policy Statement and Management Guidelines.

National Confidential Enquiry into Patient Outcome and Death (2007). *Trauma: Who Cares?* NCEPOD, London.

Airway injuries

Introduction

Life-threatening airway injuries are very rare. However, it is important to be aware that they are significantly more frequent in those sports in which blunt or crush trauma can occur, e.g. a clothes-line tackle in rugby, or blows from the fists or feet in martial art disciplines, or those that involve high speed projectiles, e.g. hockey (stick or ball).

What constitutes an airway injury?

Airway injury can potentially occur at any point in the respiratory tract. However, there are 2 key zones particularly at risk:

Face (oral and nasal cavities)

- Soft tissue swelling may result in immediate or delayed airway obstruction
- The tissues have a rich blood supply therefore persistent bleeding puts airway at risk of occlusion, e.g. severe epistaxis
- Fractures of the facial bones (nose, zygoma, maxilla, and mandible) can result in distortion of normal anatomy and encroachment on the airway, particularly when grossly displaced; they are also associated with significant bleeding that is difficult to control
- In bilateral fractures of the mandible the anterior segment has the potential to shift backwards, causing the tongue to block the airway (see 📖 p.146).

Neck (larynx and trachea)

- Soft tissue swelling with or without cartilaginous fractures can result in obstruction.
- Fractures of the larynx can occur, leading to rapid distortion of the airway and associated bleeding resulting in partial or complete airway obstruction.
- Recurrent laryngeal nerve injury may lead to vocal cord dysfunction or paralysis.

In any neck injury it is necessary to consider the possibility of a cervical cord injury or damage to the carotid vessels such as a dissection—often presenting with a history of neck injury and neurological symptoms.

How might an airway injury present?

Facial soft tissue trauma, with associated bleeding and swelling, is usually easy to recognize. If an injury is not immediately apparent, suspect airway trauma in a player complaining of:

- Dyspnoea
- Hoarseness
- Neck pain or laryngeal tenderness
- Haemoptysis
- Difficulty or pain on swallowing or talking
- Stridor—harsh inspiratory noise.

If there is immediate or impending loss of airway the player will be extremely agitated and in respiratory distress, making intervention very difficult. It is unlikely they will be co-operative! Invariably the player will become rapidly cyanosed and unconscious if the airway is not restored.

If the player is unconscious, indicators of potential airway compromise include:

- Abnormal, high-pitched inspiratory, or expiratory sounds (stridor/stertor)
- Epistaxis
- Haematoma or bruising
- Neck swelling or subcutaneous emphysema
- Loss of anatomical landmarks and/or bony crepitus (suspect an acute fracture).

:☠: **Managing airway injuries**

As with any trauma patient, a systematic assessing airway, breathing, and adequacy of circulation (A, B, C) approach should be followed along with c-spine immobilization (spinal injuries often co-exist with airway trauma). Supplementary high flow oxygen should also be administered via a non rebreathable reservoir mask.

'Walking wounded' players with a suspected airway injury should be immediately withdrawn from play. It is crucial to appreciate that the onset of signs and symptoms may be delayed and progressive, therefore loss of patency of the airway may occur precipitously. A single examination is not sufficient.

A player who may have sustained a facial fracture or has persistent epistaxis despite first line interventions (e.g. direct sustained pressure, ice application, nasal packing, and topical adrenaline) should be referred to hospital for further assessment.

Basic manoeuvre

Jaw thrust

Fingers are placed behind the angle of the jaw and the jaw is drawn forward away from the face, allowing soft tissues to be pulled away from the back of the throat (see 📖 p.23).

Airway adjuncts

(Only if patient unconscious or gag reflex is absent, e.g. GCS <8.)
- Nasopharyngeal (NP) airway (avoid if suspicion of basal skull fracture or there is nasal deformity and/or heavy bleeding):
  - Size estimation roughly by diameter of player's little finger
  - Lubricate tip, then insert with bevel facing inwards, parallel to palate, rotating gently as it is advanced.
- Oropharyngeal (OP) airway:
  - Size from angle of mandible to incisors
  - Insert with concave surface upwards, then rotate 180° once soft plate encountered or under direct vision using a torch and tongue depressor.

Advanced airway management

This requires specialist equipment and training in its use:
- *Laryngeal mask airway (LMA):* technically easy to insert, but doesn't protect from aspiration of stomach contents
- *Endo-tracheal (ET) intubation:* ideally whilst maintaining in-line immobilization.

Attempting to insert a more definitive airway should not delay transfer to hospital if basic techniques are permitting adequate gas exchange.

Surgical airway techniques

Often a last resort, but may be the only option remaining if the airway compromise is not corrected by the methods described above. Again, requires specific training and a degree of expertise.

- *Percutaneous needle cricothyroidotomy:*
  - Large bore cannula inserted into trachea though the cricothyroid membrane; oxygen tubing then attached with either a small hole made in it or 3-way valve attached
  - Allow expansion of lungs with 1 s flow on, then deflation with 4 s of flow off
  - Permits oxygenation, not ventilation, therefore CO_2 retention occurs rapidly.
- *Surgical cricothyroidotomy:* commercially available kits, e.g. Portex Minitrach II®. Permits ventilation, either spontaneously or artificially with bag and valve apparatus.

Maxillofacial injuries and infection in sports medicine

Introduction

> My face is so pretty, you don't see a scar, which proves I'm the king of the ring by far (Muhammed Ali).

Maxillofacial soft tissue and bony injuries are very common in athletes despite the recommended use of dental guards and face shields in contact sports, such as rugby and soccer. The rise in participation of contact sports, coupled with increasing pressure on individuals to maintain cosmetic appearances, have resulted in rising public perception of physical beauty demanding no imperfection, and so it is important that patients with disfiguring injuries are treated to obtain the best possible outcome both anatomically and cosmetically.

- The treating physician must be at the forefront of up-to-date management of maxillofacial injuries and infections sustained during sporting activity
- Maxillofacial injuries sustained by sportsmen (and women) vary from simple cuts and abrasions to dental injuries and severe facial fractures requiring life-saving airway support measures, and subsequent surgical fixation
- The ABC with cervical spine control assessment (as detailed in 📖 Chapter 2) must be used in all patients with maxillofacial injuries, as they are often associated with head and cervical spine injury
- The mechanism of maxillofacial injuries is generally direct impact from an external source (another player, sports equipment, the local environment, or hard surfaces)
- Forces exerted during such injuries can lead to shear, compression, friction, or traction of the soft tissues and associated structures.

⚠ As with all injuries and infection, it is assumed that the reader will perform thorough wound cleaning in extensive or heavily contaminated wounds, and human tetanus immunoglobulin (HATI) in tetanus prone wounds, and as such this will not be discussed further in this chapter.

Anatomy

- The anterior aspect of the face is bordered superiorly by the frontal bones, laterally by the temporal bones, and inferiorly by the muscles of the neck
- The facial skeleton consists of nine bones: four paired (nasal, zygomatic, maxilla, palatine, and the mandible)
- The nasal bones and zygomatic arches are prominent facial features, and, therefore, most commonly injured during facial trauma
- The nasal, frontal, and maxillary sinuses form part of the facial skeleton, and are also easily damaged in facial trauma due to being thin walled
- Motor innervation of the face is by the five main branches of the facial nerve (CN VII) as it traverses through the parotid gland, and sensory innervation by the three branches of the trigeminal nerve (CN V) The infra-orbital nerve (CN V^2) passes through the infra-orbital foramen and supplies the skin on the lateral side of the nose, the upper lip, the lower eyelid, and damage to this nerve is a good indicator of underlying zygomatico-orbital fractures.

Principles of managing maxillofacial injuries

History
- Obtain details of the mechanism of injury
- Was the athlete unconscious?
- Can they remember what happened?
- Complaints of pain, altered vision and paraesthesia must be clearly documented at the outset
- This will allow a focused assessment and may tie pathologies together such as the diplopia and cheek numbness found in an infra-orbital fracture
- In addition, a targeted medical, drug, and tetanus vaccination history should be taken, and drug allergies noted. Being aware of the athlete's past history prior to an injury occurring saves time and distraction.

Examination
- Initially assessed with the airway, breathing, circulation (ABC) approach and the cervical spine must not be overlooked—see 📖 Chapter 2
- Ensure that the airway is secure and safe before proceeding to examine injuries, and if there is any indication of immediate or potential airway compromise, seek advice and support from a colleague who can manage the airway as a matter of urgency—📖 see p.129
- The face is extremely vascular and even minor injuries may result in significant bleeding, which need to be treated quickly with irrigation and haemostatic measures (local compression or sutures) to enable thorough examination of the wound
- Initial visual inspection must take into account facial asymmetry from the front, side, and skyline views of the face. Palpate superiorly, from the frontal bones and proceed inferiorly and laterally, feeling for bony steps or crepitus
- Always examine the oral cavity for soft tissue, bony, and dental injuries, which may not be apparent externally

▶▶Document all missing and damaged teeth, and their whereabouts—if necessary you will need to ensure they are not located in the airway
- Note all areas of swelling, as this may indicate underlying injury
- The size, shape, location, and depth of lacerations needs to be clearly documented, and all wounds must be explored to exclude a foreign body (this may need to be performed under general anaesthetic, depending on the severity and complexity of the wound)
- Finally a systematic assessment of motor and sensory function of the cranial nerves supplying the face must be carried out to investigate whether there is associated nerve damage, which may require urgent repair. This is especially important in those with injuries potentially involving the facial nerve (Table 11.1) or the orbital area affecting the trigeminal nerve.

Table 11.1 Rapid assessment of facial nerve motor function

Facial nerve branch	Test of motor function
Frontalis	Look up/frown
Zygomatico-temporal	Screw up eyes
Buccal	Twitch nose
Mandibular and cervical	Purse the lips

! Soft tissue injuries

Abrasions
- Need to be thoroughly cleaned and all debris removed. Use a toothbrush if necessary to reduce the risk of infection and 'tattooing', particularly prevalent if the injury is due to contact with a tarmacadam or gravel surface
- Depending on the extent of injury this may need to be performed in the Emergency Department or even in the theatre in extensive injuries. Topical local anaesthetic in the form of lignocaine, adrenaline, and tetracaine (LAT) gel is useful here.

Haematomas
- Painful, but the vast majority will settle over a few days without intervention
- Be wary of expanding haematomas in locations that may compromise the airway or pulsatile haematomas overlying vascular structures, such as the temporal artery
- These will need review to exclude underlying vascular injury, such as a false aneurysm
- In these rare circumstances of progressive swelling overlying a blood vessel, do not aspirate, but compress and refer to hospital.

Subperichondral haematomas to the ear, often caused by blunt injury, may cause a cartilage deformity known as 'cauliflower ear'.
- This should be treated with fine needle aspiration or small incision followed by a compression dressing
- This management can be delayed until the end of the match but can be managed thereafter and the sooner the better
- Depending on experience this may be possible to perform in a sterile environment in or around the changing facilities—if in doubt refer to the hospital for formal treatment.

Lacerations
- Clean all wounds to minimize contamination and explore for foreign bodies prior to closure
- Depending on the location and size of the wound, formal closure may be delayed until after the match, i.e. eyebrow
- If in doubt obtain soft tissue X-rays for glass or metal contaminated wounds
- Simple lacerations can be closed with 5.0 or 6.0 nylon sutures. Due to the very vascular nature of the face, most lacerations tend to heal very well
- Very deep wounds, those with complicated irregular margins, or on delicate areas of the face should be referred to the appropriate specialty for formal closure
- Missed foreign bodies will usually result in infected wounds or wounds that fail to heal. If X-ray is normal then ultrasound at a later date can be useful.

Eye

- Simply asking the athlete if he can see ok is a highly useful starting point
- Ask about blurring of vision and diplopia, and check both pupils are reacting normally with no blood in the anterior chamber (hyphaema)
- Are the eye movements normal?
- Remember the assessment is about ensuring normal eye function
- The eyeball should also be fully examined for penetrating injuries, and an assessment of visual acuity, and CN II-IV and VI-VII is mandatory
- Any penetrating injury, damage to the tarsal plates, eyelid margins, lacrimal system, or the canthi should be referred to ophthalmology for further management
- Those individuals with nerve damage should be referred to the maxillofacial or plastic surgical teams for microsurgical repair
- Lacerations involving the eyebrow should be closed by alignment of the brow borders by a clinician experienced enough to manage the wound
- Do not shave eyebrow hair at wound edges as its re-growth is unpredictable. Simple eyelid lacerations can be closed as outlined above.

Mouth

- Lip lacerations involving the vermilion border should be carefully closed, as a 1-mm step in the vermilion border is visible at conversational distances
- Only carry out this procedure if you are familiar with the techniques involved—this can be done in a sterile environment in or around the changing facilities if required
- Simple intra-oral lacerations that are not full thickness should be managed by oral hygiene measures and do not require formal closure
- Full thickness intra-oral lesions that extend through to the external skin may be managed by suturing the external skin wound, leaving the intra-oral wound to heal by secondary intention with good oral hygiene
- Larger, full thickness, penetrating wounds should be referred for formal closure
- Intra-oral or full thickness wounds involving the mid-cheek should be carefully examined for parotid duct damage, as this may require referral for stenting or repair.
- Tongue lacerations will generally heal with good hygiene and do not require closure
- However, full thickness anterior lacerations, which involve the margins of the tongue, may result in a bifid tongue, so will require referral for specialist repair.

⊙ Dental injuries

- Contact sports can result in significant dental injury, which may or may not be associated with soft tissue injury and facial fractures
- Teeth can be fractured, mobilized (loosened), subluxed, or avulsed
- If possible, ask the patient to run their tongue over their teeth and check for new chips or missing teeth
- Missing teeth and fragments must be located, if not with the patient
- Ensure that associated soft tissue injuries are explored for teeth and fragments, and if necessary perform a chest X-ray to exclude the possibility of inhalation
- If you can feel or see steps in-between the teeth suspect an underlying maxillary or mandibular injury.

Fractured teeth

Do not require emergency medical management, but may cause significant pain due to exposure of the dentine, pulp, and dental nerve. Mobilized or subluxed teeth should be gently put back into normal position when possible, and then splinted appropriately.

Displaced teeth

Must be gently manipulated back into the correct position and then splinted pending urgent dental assessment. In children where only the milk teeth are involved reassurance should be given to the parents.

Avulsed teeth

- If brought in with the patient, should be gently cleaned with saline or water to remove debris—care should be taken to hold the tooth by the crown, as damaging the periodontal ligament remnants on the roots will discourage successful re-implantation
- The socket should be gently irrigated, and the tooth slowly, but firmly re-implanted (if possible) until it sits in alignment with the other teeth
- The patient must then bite down on swabs for at least half an hour
- If the tooth cannot be re-implanted (e.g. if there is associated mandibular fracture or the alveolus is damaged), it must be immersed in milk, cool tap water, or isotonic saline pending repair
- If the patient is able, the tooth can also be placed in the buccal vestibule of the mouth, between the cheek and gums, whilst en route to a dentist.

Dentoalveolar injuries

- This involves fracture of the bone and associated teeth, and must be treated as an open fracture
- Consider tetanus prophylaxis and antibiotic cover
- All dental injuries will require urgent dental review by the athlete's own dentist
- Dental injuries in association with alveolar and mandibular fractures need to be referred to the maxillofacial surgeons for appropriate immediate treatment.

:O: Maxillofacial fractures

The most common fractures in sporting injuries are of the nasal, zygomatic, orbital, and mandibular bones. Less commonly the frontal and maxillary bones will be affected when there have been high velocity injuries.

Nasal fractures

- The most common injury to the face
- The patient may have uni- or bilateral epistaxis, which may require haemostatic measures from external compression to posterior nasal packing using nasal tampons or balloon catheters
- External compression will resolve most bleeding at the pitchside:
  - If it has not subsided in under a couple of minutes then a nasal tampon is a useful second step, but effectively prevents the athlete from returning to competition in most sporting situations
  - If the bleeding is controlled pitchside and the athlete returns to play then at the end of the play examine the nose, ideally with a nasal speculum and a light source, or even an auroscope in the dressing room
  - In patients with nasal injuries, those with a septal haematoma may progress to cartilage necrosis if this is not drained over the next 12–24 h. A septal haematoma resembles a blue-red swelling originating from the septum.
- Fractures can be referred to Ear, Nose, and Throat (ENT) department after 5–7 days, allowing the swelling to settle so the extent of the fracture can be fully assessed
- At that point, any significant cosmetic deformity or nasal airway defect can be surgically corrected
- Do not delay further as operative fixation will be hampered by any delay more than 7 days
- Cerebrospinal fluid (CSF) rhinorrhoea, often seen as a 'tramline' of blood, edged by clear fluid indicates damage to the naso-ethmoidal area and warrants urgent CT imaging (see 📖 p.113).

Zygomatic (cheekbone) fractures

- Patient may have significant swelling over the flattened zygomatic bone
- Those with lateral and inferior orbital wall damage may have altered infra-orbital nerve sensation, peri-orbital haematoma, subconjunctival haemorrhage, diplopia, and restriction of eye movements superiorly (3rd nerve entrapment)
- Those with fractures involving the zygomatic arch may have restricted mouth opening due to the depressed arch impinging on the temporalis muscle, where it inserts on the mandibular coronoid process
- Occipitomental and sub-mentovertex facial X-rays will allow confirmation of a fracture and associated displacement
- Zygomatic fractures should be referred immediately to the maxillofacial surgeons for review and possible operative fixation.

Orbital (blow out) fractures

- Involve the orbital floor and the medial wall, and are usually associated with significant peri-orbital swelling and ecchymosis
- The infra-orbital nerve may be damaged causing paraesthesia over the infra-orbital area, and tethering of the muscles of the eye causing loss of upward movement of the eye and subsequent diplopia
- These signs may occur together or in isolation, and are individually suggestive of a fracture. Enopthalmos may be seen
- Facial X-rays may show the classic 'teardrop' sign, indicating the prolapse of the herniated orbital contents (peri-orbital fat and the inferior rectus muscle) through the orbital floor into the maxillary sinus
- However, if normal, but with persistent symptoms then CT scan of the orbital floor is a far more sensitive investigation.

⚠ A child presenting with signs of an inferior rectus muscle entrapment, such as diplopia on upwards gaze should have this surgically decompressed emergently by a facial specialist in theatre due to the risk of muscle necrosis. This pathology differs from the adult where there is no such trap-door effect and thus may be managed less urgently.

Mandibular fractures

- Due to the horseshoe structure of the mandible, fractures are generally bilateral and often occur at its weakest points—the condylar neck, the angle of the jaw, and the distal body
- The patient may present with malocclusion, pain, and swelling around the jaw, difficulty mouth opening, intra-oral bleeding and paraesthesia of the ipsilateral lower lip due to mandibular nerve damage
- The mandible may be deviated to one side, and intra-oral examination may reveal a palpable bony step of the dental margins
- Orthopantomogram (OPT) and mandibular X-rays will reveal the site of a mandibular fracture
- Bilateral or open fractures require IV antibiotic prophylaxis and referral to the maxillofacial surgeons for repair.

Mandibular dislocation

- This can occur uni- and bilaterally, and presents with the mouth hanging open and the patient drooling
- Palpating the temporomandibular joints may reveal swelling and tenderness
- In an athlete with recurrent dislocations, relocation can be performed pitchside by standing in front of the patient and applying slow, but firm manual pressure (protect your fingers by placing swabs on the teeth) bilaterally to the molars in an infero-posterior direction
- In an athlete presenting for the first time then this should not be attempted pitchside and referral to hospital for X-ray to ensure no associated fracture.

Maxillary fractures

- Are not commonly seen during sporting injuries
- They are commonly caused by high velocity blunt impact, and must be excluded when there is dental malocclusion present
- The patient may have associated airway disruption, and this must be secured before assessing the extent of these fractures by CT.

There are three main types of maxillary fracture according to the Le For classification system (Table 11.2).

Table 11.2 Le Fort classification of maxillary fractures

Le Fort Classification	Fracture and margins
I	Horizontal, extending from nasal septum to pterygoid plates
II	Pyramidal, extending from nasal bone down to pterygoid plates
III	Transverse, extending from nasal sinuses to pterygoid plates

Frontal bone fracture

- The supraorbital margins may be disrupted, and subcutaneous emphysema may be palpated
- Check the function of the superior orbital and trochlear nerves. Suspect a dural tear in extensive frontal injuries, which may involve fractures of the posterior wall of the frontal bone
- These fractures are often associated with polytrauma, and require physiological stability before CT imaging and definitive management.

✛ Medical maxillofacial emergencies

The skin

Cellulitis
- Occurs around a site of trauma
- Causes erythema and swelling of the skin
- Oral antibiotics to treat common skin bacteria (*Staph. aureus* and *Staph. pyogenes*) are suitable for most cases
- However, peri-orbital cellulitis must be treated with high dose IV antibiotics to avoid spread into the orbital area so referral is required.

Spots and lesions
- If affecting the nasal area (the so-called 'danger area' of the face) can migrate posteriorly via the ophthalmic veins, causing haematological spread of infection into the cavernous sinus and can cause meningitis, or cerebral abscesses
- Patients will present with an obvious nasal region infection, and may have a pyrexia, confusion, and headache
- Treat with analgesia and antibiotics, and refer for specialist assessment.

Herpes zoster virus infection ('shingles')
A very painful skin infection, forming vesicles in the distribution of one dermatome. It results from reactivation of Varicella zoster in patients previously exposed. It is treated with analgesia and oral acyclovir.

Patients with ophthalmic shingles should be carefully monitored and referred to an ophthalmologist to avoid eye involvement.

Herpes gladiatorum ('scrumpox')
- A skin infection caused by the herpes simplex virus, and occurs following skin-to-skin (often stubble to face) contact, e.g. during a rugby scrum
- It is characterized by clusters of fluid filled blisters, which are painful
- Treatment consists of good hygiene, not sharing towels, excluding affected players until symptoms cease, analgesia, and acyclovir
- Scrumpox may be impetiginous and caused by *Staph. aureus* or *Staph. pyogenes*, and require antibiotic therapy
- Occasionally *Tinea barbae* may be the causative organism requiring treatment with anti-fungals.

Actinomycosis
- Caused by the bacterium *Actinomyces israelii*. It occurs in golfers who put golf tees in their mouth during play, and causes dental abscesses and sinusitis
- There is usually an underlying concurrent dental problem—poor dental hygiene or recent dental work
- Once in the tissues, it may also cause hard reddish purple skin lumps, that progress to form purulent discharging abscesses
- Treatment is long term, with up to 4 weeks of IV penicillin and several months of oral therapy. It may also be necessary to surgically drain abscesses and sinuses.

The eye

Conjunctivitis

- Viral or bacterial in origin, this can affect one or both eyes
- The patient will complain of red, gritty eyes with increased tearing
- Full eye examination must be performed to exclude foreign bodies or ulceration on the cornea
- Treatment should include analgesia, and topical chloramphenicol applied for 5 days.

Acanthoemoebic keratitis

- A water-borne infection, which can cause pain, keratitis, and ulceration in watersports participants
- Especially common in swimmers who wear contact lens in the pool
- Treatment is with analgesia and corneal debridement, followed by antimicrobial therapy.

The mouth

Toothache

- Caused by dental caries, broken fillings, and dental abscesses
- Symptoms include throbbing dental pain, headache, altered taste, and sensitivity to foods and temperature
- Treatment with anti-inflammatories is recommended, and if there is evidence of a swelling around a dental root then a 1-week course of antibiotics should be prescribed to treat dental abscess
- Such patients should be referred to their dentist for repair of caries or abscess incision and drainage.

Wisdom teeth (third molars) usually develop between the ages of 18–25 years old.

- They are normal teeth and do not need to be extracted unless they cause problems
- Impaction of the wisdom teeth occurs due to lack of space meaning they only partly come through the gums
- They can be associated with infection due to gum tissue that can sit on top of the teeth allowing food and bacteria to build up underneath and abscesses to subsequently develop
- Infections should be treated with antibiotics and dental review
- Certain types of impaction can cause weakness to the mandible and be associated with an increased incidence of mandibular fractures
- The problematic wisdom teeth can be extracted depending on a number of factors, such as the degree of impaction and the age of the patient
- Depending on how many need to be removed and their position they can be removed under local anaesthetic with or without sedation, or in hospital as part of a general anaesthetic
- If 'elective' then extraction should be undertaken during the off-season
- Return to light training can be between 7–10 days and return to contact sport usually 2–3 weeks depending on the complexity of the surgery.

Ulcers
- Breach in the oral mucosa exposing the underlying connective tissue
- Commonly caused by infection or trauma, these lesions are extremely painful, and should be treated with analgesia and chlorhexidine or salt mouthwashes
- Persistent oral ulceration should raise suspicion of underlying malignancy or systemic conditions, e.g. Aphthous ulceration in Crohn's disease, and refer to a specialist for investigation.

Herpes simplex virus
- Clinically manifests as 'cold sores' on the lips
- It initially presents with a burning tingling sensation before the appearance of crops of golden vesicles
- It can be treated with acyclovir, but the mainstay of treatment is good hygiene between players to avoid spread.

The sinuses

Sinusitis
- Results from infection (bacterial, viral, fungal, and allergic) or inflammation, and can cause excruciating pain
- It is associated with headaches and thick purulent nasal discharge, and can be very debilitating
- Treatment is supportive with analgesia and antibiotics if symptoms are prolonged
- Patients suffering from chronic (symptoms lasting beyond 12 weeks) or recurring sinusitis may benefit from maxillofacial referral for surgical drainage.

Spinal injuries

Introduction

- Spinal injuries may consist of bony and/or ligamentous damage with or without neurological damage. Such injuries are uncommon in sport, but certain sports carry a higher inherent risk such as rugby or eventing.

For the purposes of this chapter:
- **Spinal injuries** will refer to injuries with or without neurological deficit
- **Spinal cord injuries** refer to those injuries which present with neurological deficit
- **Primary spinal cord injury** is the injury to the cord resulting in direct compressive forces from unstable bony architecture
- **Secondary spinal cord injury** is the result of changes at a cellular level caused by factors such as hypoxia or hypovolaemia.

Any medical professional who is pitchside must be able to:
- Recognize the potential for spinal injury with and without cord damage
- Recognize that there is the potential to cause worsening of the primary injury by failing to appropriately assess and immmobilize and secure the cervical spine
- This failure may lead to spinal cord injury in a previously undamaged spinal cord or further damage to a spinal cord that was damaged at the time of the original injury (e.g. a partial cord transection becoming complete)
- Close observation of the athlete may give the clinician vital clues as to the mechanism of injury and therefore the likelihood of spinal injury. This is especially useful when the athlete may have suffered concurrent head trauma and potentially not be capable of giving an (accurate) history.

If you do not clearly witness the incident, then:
- Consider the situation, e.g. was the injury sustained during the collapse of a rugby scrum or has a gymnast fallen from a piece of apparatus?
- Make your initial assessment whilst applying manual in-line stabilization to the cervical spine
- Obtain eye witness reports where possible
- Have a low threshold for suspecting spinal injury:
  - In some circumstances, it may quickly become obvious that you are not dealing with a spinal injury
  - At other times where there may be spinal pain but you do not suspect a spinal cord injury, then a formal procedure to clear the spine clinically may be attempted.

Essential equipment and training

To manage a spinal injury pitchside, the essential equipment consists of:
- Oxygen
- Spinal board, head blocks, and straps (along with application of a cervical collar this constitutes triple immobilization)
- Cervical collars (adjustable or various sizes, including paediatric if appropriate)
- IV access, drugs, fluids for neurogenic shock.

You will need to be confident in the following procedures:
- Primary survey assessment
- Manual in-line stabilization (MILS)
- Sizing and application of a cervical collar
- Log rolling
- Transfer and securing onto a spinal board
- Safely re-positioning the athlete from their position of injury to one where they may be transferred onto a spinal board (usually this means keeping their spine straight and placing them supine
- However, if their neurological symptoms worsen as you attempt to move them or pain/muscle spasm prevents movement, then you may have to stabilize them in the position in which you found them)
- Potentially directing untrained personnel to assist you in some of the above (only if the athlete must be transferred from the field of play before paramedics are in attendance).

Note: The above points assume that there are no other injuries requiring management. There is no substitute for practice and many courses are available locally and nationally to learn the practical techniques listed above.

☠ Pitchside care of suspected spinal injury

It is important to treat all patients in a systematic fashion according to the principles of ABCDE, including a safe approach to the patient (see 📖 pp.13–14).

When you suspect a potential spinal injury, then assessment of the airway must be accompanied by manual in-line stabilization of the cervical spine. High flow oxygen should be applied immediately to help prevent secondary insult to the spinal cord.

Practical tips on airway assessment with cervical spine control

Athletes do not always fall helpfully into a supine position to enable easy assessment of their airway along with manual in-line stabilization.

- If they are not supine but you are still able to assess the airway, then stabilize them manually in the position in which you find them
- If there is any airway compromise which cannot be managed in their original position, then you will have to turn them
- Adapt the technique for log rolling, but remember the airway takes priority over potential spinal cord damage. If they are not breathing sufficiently to achieve adequate oxygenation, you may have to turn whilst maintaining what stabilizing forces around the spine possible
- If someone with airway compromise has a suspected cervical spine injury, a jaw thrust (not head tilt/chin lift) should be used to open the airway
- Manual in-line immobilization (MILS) may be adapted to provide jaw thrust concurrently should airway support be required (if persistent jaw thrust is required, you may want to consider an adjunct airway).

The following is a stepwise approach to the assessment and management of a suspected spinal injury pitchside:

- SAFE approach and call for assistance as the scene dictates
- Immediately apply manual in line immobilization and assess the airway.
  - Can the patient talk to you?
  - If possible, obtain a history from the athlete, especially regarding spinal pain and neurological symptoms. (Turning the athlete into a supine position may be required to assess and/or manage the airway adequately)
- Ask someone to call 999 for paramedic assistance (if they are not already in attendance)—ask them to tell the operator that you are dealing with a suspected spinal cord injury and get them to come back and confirm that they are on their way
- Continue with MILS, until triple immobilization is complete.
- This consists of:
  - Correctly-sized semi-rigid collar applied correctly
  - Head blocks or equivalent
  - Tape or straps placed over the forehead and blocks, attached to the extraction device, together with a second tape or strap over the chin
- Assessment of breathing and circulation (see 📖 pp.13–14 for details) and manage issues with ABC as they arise (see 📖 earlier chapters for details)

- Administer high flow oxygen
- Briefly assess disability:
  - AVPU or GCS (GCS; see 📖 p.116)
  - Active movement in all 4 limbs
  - Sensation to light touch in hands and feet
  - If there is any neurological deficit then assume a cord injury and manage accordingly
- Log roll onto the spinal board (see 📖 p.15 for details). Continue to apply manual in-line stabilization throughout this as the collar only reduces cervical movement by about 30%
- Put the head blocks in place and apply the straps or tape
- Continuously reassess ABC's and monitor for changes in neurology during the above
- Arrange transfer to the nearest Emergency Department (ED) capable of dealing with spinal injuries such as a major trauma centre. Depending on the condition of the athlete and your other responsibilities you may wish to accompany them.

Clinical practice tips regarding athlete extraction

- Whenever you are working in a new location or with a new team then aim to have a run through of how you would extract an athlete with a suspected cord injury before the competition starts.
- Make sure everyone (clinical and non-clinical) know their roles e.g. fetching equipment, assisting with log roll, calling the paramedics.

Note: The procedure is exactly the same for an athlete with a thoracic or lumbar spinal injury—the neck should still be immobilized as part of the triple immobilization.

☼ 'Clearing' the cervical spine

You may be called to see an athlete who has gone down and is complaining of neck pain, but in whom you think a spinal injury is unlikely. For example, a clash of heads on the football pitch and on assessment the athlete is fully alert, has no signs of a head injury, and is complaining of mild pain on one side of their neck.

- In such a scenario you may attempt to clear the cervical spine clinically.
- The starting point always remains the same, i.e. inline stabilization whilst assessing ABC.
- If ABCs are normal, then you may clear the spine clinically if ALL of the following criteria are met (based on NEXUS low risk criteria; Panacek et al. 2001):
  - (1) GCS 15/15 (and no evidence of intoxication)
  - (2) No distracting injury, e.g. ankle fracture dislocation
  - (3) No neurological deficit (moving all 4 limbs, normal sensation, not complaining of paraesthesia)
  - (4) No posterior midline cervical tenderness—ask someone else to stabilize the neck from the front whilst you palpate the spine
- If all the above are met then proceed to active movements as a final check (based on Canadian C-spine Rule; Stiell et al. 2003):
  - (5) Ask the athlete to gently rotate their head in a lateral direction, first one way then the next. Continue to support the head, but ensure the movements are active (i.e. the athlete is moving his neck not you!) and not passive. There should be 45° of lateral rotation in both directions without significant pain
  - (6) No concern over the mechanism of injury, i.e. after a fall from a horse you should have a very low thresh-hold of suspecting spinal injury even if steps 1–5 are clear
- If the athlete successfully progresses through the NEXUS criteria then release manual in-line stabilization and gently sit them up
- If they can take the weight of their head and move their neck reasonably comfortably then they can be managed as for a soft tissue injury
- If at any stage they fail a criterion or if the mechanism of injury is a concern then transfer to nearest appropriate ED.

✪ Recognizing neurological signs

The conscious patient may complain of:
- Inability to move limbs
- Loss of sensation
- Altered sensation
- Burning pain in the limbs
- A mixture of all or some of the above.

A number of 'incomplete' cord syndromes have been described relating to the neurology signs that will be demonstrated depending on which aspect of the cord has been injured.

Central cord syndrome
- Usually results from falling directly onto the face resulting in a hyperextension injury
- Characterized by disproportionately greater motor loss in the upper extremities compared with the lower extremities—'able to walk but not move arms'
- Variable degree of sensory loss below the level of injury
- Incomplete cord injury.

Brown sequard
- Usually result of penetrating trauma
- Hemisection of the cord
- Motor loss and numbness to touch and vibration on the same side of the spinal injury
- Loss of pain and temperature sensation on the opposite side.

Anterior cord syndrome
- Partial spinal cord injury
- Often vascular in origin
- Complete muscle paralysis below the level of the injury with loss of pain and temperature sensation
- Proprioception and vibration sensation is not affected.

Complications of cord injury

The level of the injury may affect the patient's breathing.

C1–2
- Inability to breathe due to intercostal and diaphragmatic paralysis
- Requires immediate breathing support to survive.

C3–5
- Phrenic nerve may be involved leading to difficulty breathing
- Even if a patient is able to breathe, initially they will tire easily and need close monitoring.

C5–7
Seesaw respiratory pattern due to paralysis of intercostal muscles, but functioning diaphragm.

T1–L2
- Variable loss of intercostal muscle function and thus respiratory function
- The anatomical level of the primary injury may be falsely reassuring in that haematoma and swelling may be found 1–2 vertebral bodies more proximally than the level found on initial examination or imaging
- The pitchside doctor will need to treat all spinal injury patients with high flow oxygen and may need to provide respiratory support with a bag valve mask.

✪ Cord injury and shock

▶▶ Initial management should include thorough and repeated assessment to ensure you do not miss an alternative cause for hypotension. (see Chapter 2).

Neurogenic shock/bradyarrhythmia

In those with cervical or upper thoracic cord injuries, the sympathetic chain may be damaged, leading to parasympathetic activity being unchecked.

- The patient will be 'warm and hypotensive' with bradyarrhythmia or even asystole
- Atropine can be used to treat bradycardia, (although this would not necessarily be expected as part of the standard pitchside drug bag)
- Ensure adequate oxygenation and enable rapid paramedic assistance and transfer to nearest ED if the athlete is showing signs of bradycardia
- IV fluids, e.g. normal saline may be administered to maintain a systolic blood pressure (BP) of 80–90 mmHg. There is a risk that chasing the BP with fluids will result in fluid overload and vasopressors may be required instead in the ED (It is, however, unlikely that fluid overload will be an issue in the pre-hospital setting)
- Beware of other causes of hypotension (e.g. from hypovolaemia, suggesting internal bleeding). If the shock is hypovolaemic, usually the pulse rate will be raised. Remember, however, the two forms of shock may co-exist and the key to managing these patients is regular repeated assessments.

Spinal shock

- This is not shock as classically defined in terms of a failure to perfuse vital organs
- It refers to the immediate loss of reflexes and flaccidity seen after cord injury with subsequent return of hyper-reflexia found weeks after the injury
- Spinal shock and neurogenic shock are not interchangeable terms.

① Back pain associated with acute disc prolapse

Consider this in any sudden onset of acute back pain. The radiation of the pain will depend on the level of the disc affected. For example, cervical discs will radiate into the shoulders and arms, while lumbar discs will give pain radiating into the legs. The radiation of the pain occurs due to irritation of the nerve roots, rather than the cord and will give unilateral signs and symptoms.

- Initial treatment will be analgesia and, if associated with trauma, immobilization
- Neurological examination should identify the level of the disc affected.

Cauda equina syndrome

- Central disc herniation at L4–5 level below the end of the spinal cord (i.e. below L2/3)
- Severe pain
- Loss of peri-anal sensation due to involvement of S1–2 with saddle anaesthesia and decreased anal tone
- Loss of ability to control micturition with urinary retention
- This requires immediate referral for decompression.

▶▶ Remember that in patients over the age of 50 presenting with a traumatic back pain, the diagnosis of other conditions, such as an aortic aneurysm should be considered and abdominal examination carried out.

Further reading

Blackmore, C.C. (2003). Evidence-based imaging evaluation of the cervical spine in trauma. *Neuroimaging Clin N Am* **13**(2): 283–91.

Hoffman, J.R., Wolfson, A.B., Todd, K., Mower, W.R. (1998). Selective cervical spine radiography in blunt trauma: methodology of the National Emergency X-Radiography Utilization Study (NEXUS). *Ann Emerg Med* **32**(4): 461–9.

Panacek, E.A., Mower, W.R., Holmes, J.F., Hoffman, J.R. (2001). NEXUS group. Test performance of the individual NEXUS low-risk clinical screening criteria for cervical spine injury. *Ann Emerg Med* **38**(1): 22–5.

Stiell, I.G., Clement, C.M., McKnight, R.D., et al. (2003). The Canadian C-spine rule versus the NEXUS low-risk criteria in patients with trauma. *N Engl J Med* **349**(26): 2510–18.

Vinson, D.R. (2001). NEXUS cervical spine criteria. *Ann Emerg Med* **37**(2): 237–8.

Thorax

Introduction

Medical conditions or trauma involving the chest during sport and exercise are a rare but a potentially serious problem.

Although exercise itself, or the environment in which we exercise, can exacerbate underlying medical conditions such as asthma, the more common chest-related problems in sports are those involving trauma.

- Impairment can be as a result of blunt (such as a closed compression mechanism) or penetrating trauma
- The more severe injuries are usually as a consequence of a high velocity impact, such as is seen in motor racing
- However, chest injuries can occur in any contact sport or where there is a fall at speed or from a height, and these can ultimately be as potentially severe.

Anatomy

- The chest wall comprises of 12 pairs of ribs and the two layers of intercostal muscles that lie between them
- Beneath each rib lies the neurovascular bundle, containing an intercostal nerve, artery, and vein
- All the ribs are attached posteriorly to the 12 thoracic vertebrae. The first seven pairs of ribs articulate anteriorly with the sternum via the costochondral cartilages
- The following three pairs share a common cartilaginous connection to the sternum, whereas the last two pairs (eleventh and twelfth ribs) have no connection with the sternum and are termed *floating ribs*
- The sternum in turn articulates with the clavicles via synovial joints
- The chest cavity is separated from the abdomen by the muscular diaphragm, which can rise to the level of the fourth intercostal space during full expiration
- It is therefore essential that when assessing a chest injury, we are aware of the possibility of an underlying abdominal injury
- Abdominal viscera particularly at risk are the spleen, the liver, and the kidneys.

Preparation and risk management

It is essential that detailed preparation is undertaken prior to any sporting activity. Essential information required particularly relating to chest conditions would include:

- *Past medical history:* particularly any underlying lung or heart conditions
- *Relevant medications:* their requirements before, during, and after exercise and their relevance with the World Anti-Doping Agency
- *Any recent chest injuries:* as a graduated rehabilitation and return to contact sports may be required
- A concise knowledge of the environment in which the activity is to take place (see 📕 Chapter 6).

Standard medical equipment

- This should relate to the activity, potential injuries, and environment
- Appropriate protective equipment should be used depending on the sport, e.g. chest and spine protectors
- Appropriate sport-specific training and fitness testing, with adequate rest and staged return after injury and illness.

⚙ Trauma

Any assessment of the chest after trauma must first include an assessment of the airway and consideration of a cervical spine injury.

Assessment of patient

The patient's chest, back, and neck must be fully exposed. Injuries and respiratory or circulatory compromise can be identified by:

- *Looking:*
  - Respiratory rate
  - Quality and depth of breathing
  - Unequal or paradoxical chest movements
  - Use of accessory muscles
  - Central cyanosis
  - Distension of neck veins
  - Bruising and abrasions
- *Listening:*
  - Inspiratory stridor indicative of an upper airway compromise, e.g. foreign body
  - Expiratory wheeze indicative of a lower airway compromise, e.g. asthma
  - Reduced air entry
  - Abnormal chest percussion (dull or hyper-resonant)
- *Feeling:*
  - Position of trachea
  - Surgical emphysema
  - Unequal chest movements
  - Pain.

⚠ Significant internal injury to the chest can occur without an obvious external injury.

Rib fractures

- The protective framework of the upper part of the chest includes the scapula, the humerus, the clavicle, and all their muscular attachments
- Together these provide quite an extensive protective framework
- Any fracture to upper ribs (1–3) therefore suggests a magnitude of injury that places the head, spine, lungs, heart, and great vessels all at serious risk of injury
- The middle ribs (4–9) sustain the majority of blunt trauma
- Anteroposterior forces (such as a fall from a horse) generally force the ribs outwards resulting in a fracture of the midshaft of the rib
- Direct forces to the ribs, (such as elbows) generally drive them into the thorax with potential for injuries such as pneumothorax, haemothorax, or tension pneumothorax
- Fractures of the lower ribs (10–12) increase the suspicion of an associated intra-abdominal injury.

Because younger individuals have more flexible chest walls, their ribs are more likely to bend than to break.

⚠ There should therefore be a high level of suspicion of a serious associated injury in the presence of rib fractures in a child or young adult.
- Pain aggravated by deep breathing or coughing with localized tenderness or palpable crepitus over the affected rib would suggest a rib fracture
- In most cases the treatment is NSAID analgesia and rest for up to 6 weeks
- Breathing exercises are encouraged, as the pain can result in splinting of the thorax, which can impair ventilation and an effective cough
- This can lead to atelectasis and pneumonia, particularly in those who have underlying lung disease or who smoke
- Stress fractures of the ribs (most commonly the first rib) can also occur and are seen in athletes who compete in overhead sports, such as basketball or tennis
- There is no acute traumatic event, but due to the repeated contractions of the anterior scalene muscle the rib stresses and breaks
- Treatment is analgesia and rest with a graded return to full activity over 1–2 months.

Pneumothorax

A pneumothorax occurs when air accumulates in the pleural cavity, a potential space, which lies between the visceral and parietal pleura.
- This occurs either from the outside in the case of an open pneumothorax (which is rare in sport) or from the lung itself—a closed pneumothorax
- It can occur spontaneously in the absence of trauma, or as a result of a penetrating or crush injury.

Spontaneous pneumothoraces
- Can be primary or secondary:
  - Primary spontaneous pneumothoraces are more often seen in tall, thin young men without underlying lung disease. They are usually characterized by a rupture of an imperfection in the lining of the lung (bleb) causing the lung to deflate
  - Secondary pneumothoraces are as a result of underlying lung disease such as asthma, Marfan's syndrome, cystic fibrosis, infection, or carcinoma
- When a pneumothorax is present, the patient will complain of pleuritic pain, and they may be tachycardic and tachypnoic
  - Breath sounds are decreased on the affected side and the chest is hyper-resonant to percussion
  - There may be subcutaneous emphysema felt around the neck, axillae, or chest wall, but ultimately a chest X-ray is required to confirm the diagnosis
- In hospital, small traumatic pneumothoraces may be treated conservatively; however, most are safely treated with the insertion of a chest drain in the fourth or fifth intercostal space. Aspiration can be attempted, but is a more appropriate treatment for a primary spontaneous pneumothorax

⚠ A patient with a pneumothorax *should not* travel by air. Airlines currently arbitrarily advise that there should be a 6-week interval between X-ray confirmed resolution of a pneumothorax and travelling by air.

Pneumothorax and diving
Advice for return to diving is generally related to the nature of the pneumothorax. Because of the high risk of recurrence of a spontaneous pneumothorax (up to 50% in some studies) this is regarded as an absolute contra-indication to diving.

A pneumothorax secondary to trauma, however, is related to a specific injury that if fully healed should not predispose the pleura to risk of a further pneumothorax. In this situation, a normal clinical examination and CT scan is advised to show full healing of any rib fractures and full expansion of the lung prior to return to diving.

⚠ Tension pneumothorax

This is a life-threatening emergency and requires prompt recognition and treatment. As a result of a one-way valve leak, the air in the pleural cavity continues to accumulate. The resulting increase in the intrathoracic pressure gives rise to mediastinal shift and an increasing pressure on the interthoracic vessels. This leads to a reduction in venous return to the heart, and thus a decreased cardiac output resulting in profound hypotension and death if left untreated.

⚠ A tension pneumothorax is a clinical diagnosis based on the diagnosis of a pneumothorax associated with signs of shock.
  Features include:
• Chest pain
• Hypotension
• Respiratory distress
• Tachycardia
• Distended neck veins
• A deviated trachea away from the affected side (although this is a rare finding)
• Hyper-resonant chest to percussion.

Treatment
• Treatment is high flow oxygen and immediate needle decompression—if appropriately trained:
  • This involves the insertion of a large bore cannula into the second intercostal space anteriorly in the mid-clavicular line
  • A loud hiss may be heard as the needle breaches the pleura and releases some of the intra-thoracic pressure (Fig. 13.1)
• This is a life-saving, but only temporary procedure as the cannula is at risk of kinking and blocking
• Regular assessment and the timely insertion of a chest drain is required.

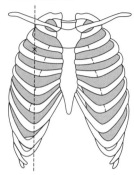

Mid-clavicular line

Fig. 13.1 Site for needle decompression of right tension pneumothorax. Reproduced from Wyatt et al., *Oxford Handbook of Emergency Medicine*, 2006, with permission from Oxford University Press.

Haemothorax

- A haemothorax is a condition that results from blood accumulating in the pleural cavity usually as a result of a lung laceration or a laceration to an intercostal or internal mammary vessels
- Its cause can be blunt or penetrating trauma and blood loss into the pleural cavity can be massive as each side of the thorax can hold 30–40% of the total circulating volume
- If left untreated it may progress to a point where the accumulating blood starts to put pressure on the mediastinum and great vessels in much the same way as a tension pneumothorax
- This together with the associated blood loss can quickly lead to profound hypotension, shock and subsequent death
- Diagnosis can be made clinically:
  - The patient will complain of pain with associated tachycardia and tachypnoea
  - Decreased or absent breath sounds on the affected side will be found in association with a chest that is dull to percussion
  - It is dullness to percussion that is one of the main clinical pointers to allow differentiation between massive haemothorax and tension pneumothorax where percussion is hyper-resonant
  - There may be additional signs of blood loss and shock depending on the size of the haemothorax
- A haemothorax is managed in the pre-hospital environment with high flow oxygen and judicious fluid replacement:
  - In the hospital setting treatment involves draining the blood already accumulated in the thoracic cavity
  - Blood in the cavity can be removed with the insertion of a chest drain and as the lung expands the bleeding will generally stop

- If the bleeding does not slow down or stop then urgent surgery will be required to temper the bleeding source.

⚠ If you have doubt about whether the athlete is suffering from tension pneumothorax or massive haemothorax, and they are peri-arrest with respiratory compromise, then there is much to be gained by decompressing the chest with a needle as described earlier. It will make little difference in the case of a massive haemothorax, but will be life-saving in tension.

Open pneumothorax
- Large defects of the chest wall, which remain open, result in an open pneumothorax
- A negative intrathoracic pressure is generated during inspiration so that air is entrained or sucked into the chest cavity through the hole in the chest wall
- If the opening in the chest wall is approximately two-thirds the diameter of the trachea, air passes preferentially through the chest defect with each breath
- The result is inadequate ventilation and a progressive buildup of air and, therefore, subsequent pressure in the pleural space
- Diagnosis should be made clinically during the primary survey
- Any wound in the chest wall that appears to be 'sucking air' into the chest or is visibly bubbling is diagnostic of an open pneumothorax
- Initial management is high flow oxygen and subsequent prompt closure of the defect with a sterile occlusive dressing taped on three sides. This produces a flutter-type valve, which allows air to pass out when the patient exhales, but gets sucked shut on inhalation preventing air from entering
- A chest drain is then required. Regular assessment is required as a dressing closed on all four sides can convert an open pneumothorax to a tension pneumothorax.

Flail segment
- A flail segment occurs as a result of multiple rib fractures, i.e. 3 or more rib fractures in 2 or more places
- The chest wall fails to move properly resulting in a paradoxical breathing pattern where the isolated area of chest wall moves inward with inspiration and outwards during expiration
- A flail chest is a high-energy injury and should prompt transfer to hospital for investigation of damage to underlying viscera (e.g. pulmonary contusion, pneumothorax, or haemothorax)
- Crepitus of rib fractures felt in an area, where the chest wall is seen to be moving paradoxically is diagnostic of a flail chest
- This is a potentially life-threatening injury and will frequently require a period of assisted ventilation. Initial treatment is to provide oxygen, analgesia, assess for other associated injuries and arrange immediate transfer to an appropriate emergency department that can continue to assess and if necessary further assist ventilation.

Cardiac tamponade

- Traumatic cardiac tamponade occurs when the pericardium fills with blood as a result of penetrating or blunt injury
- The pericardial sac is a fixed fibrous structure so only a relatively small amount of blood (~100 mL) is required to restrict cardiac contractility and reduce cardiac output
- The diagnosis can be difficult and the classic signs of hypotension, jugular venous distension, and muffled heart sounds (Beck's triad) are not always easy to elicit, especially in a noisy sporting arena
- If, however, a traumatic chest injury has occurred where there is a high index of suspicion for a cardiac tamponade and a patient is unresponsive to resuscitative efforts for hemorrhagic shock and/or a tension pneumothorax then a pericardiocentesis may be considered
- If you have been appropriately trained then this involves the removal of blood from the pericardium by a long 18G needle
- The needle is inserted 1–2 cm below the xiphisternum at 45° to the skin and advanced towards the left shoulder tip
- Aspiration of 20–30 mL of blood from the pericardium is diagnostic and may temporarily improve cardiac output until a more definitive treatment can be arranged.

Pulmonary contusion

- Pulmonary contusions are caused by a high energy, blunt trauma, and are the most common potentially lethal chest injury
- It is also commonly seen in patients with flail chest and multiple rib fractures
- The diagnosis is made radiologically in a patient who over a period of time becomes progressively short of breath and hypoxic
- Supportive measures before transfer to hospital include high flow oxygen, judicious fluids, analgesia, and appropriate monitoring.

Sternal fractures

These fractures occur as a result of direct high energy trauma. The primary significance is that it can indicate the presence of serious associated internal injuries, especially to the heart and lungs. Any athlete with a suspected fractured sternum must be assessed in hospital and will require a period of observation unless they have an isolated sternal fracture, a normal ECG and no associated injuries.

Signs and symptoms

- Crepitus
- Pain
- Tenderness
- Bruising
- Swelling over the fracture site.

The fracture may visibly move when the person breathes, and it may be bent or deformed, potentially forming a 'step' at the junction of the broken bone ends that is detectable by palpation. Associated injuries, such as those to the heart may cause symptoms, such as abnormalities seen on electrocardiograms.

The abdomen

Introduction

- Assessment of the abdomen is a key part of the initial approach to an injured or unwell athlete and should be examined as part of the evaluation of circulation
- In sport the abdominal contents may be vulnerable to sudden deceleration, blunt impact, or penetrating injury
- Bleeding from vessels/solid organs or rupture of hollow viscera can lead to hypovolaemic shock or sepsis
- In-built protection comes from the lower ribs, tensed muscles, abdominal, and retroperitoneal fat, and can be augmented by protective equipment
- Even small and initially occult internal injuries can lead to devastating shock and in a fit athlete a considerable amount of blood can be sequestered in the abdominal cavity before external signs become evident
- Damaged viscera may be difficult to detect clinically and/or masked by other injuries. A high index of suspicion and repeated examinations by the same person are necessary, with a low threshold for transfer to hospital and imaging.

Anatomy

- The anterior abdomen extends from the trans-nipple line superiorly to the inguinal ligaments, and symphysis pubis inferiorly and laterally to the anterior axillary lines, with the flanks extending as far as the posterior axillary lines
- The upper abdominal cavity, bounded by the diaphragm, lies within the thoracic cage and rises as high as the fourth intercostal space in full expiration
- The lower part of the cavity lies between the alae of the iliac bones. The vertebral column and thick back muscles lie posteriorly with thinner musculature anteriorly and laterally
- These bony relations and contraction of the muscles offer a degree of protection from injury, but trauma to the lower thorax, back, and buttocks can impact on the contents of the abdomen
- It is helpful to divide the abdomen into four quadrants for descriptive purposes and to correlate areas of local tenderness with the underlying structures (Fig. 14.1 and Table 14.1).

Knowledge of patterns of referred pain can help identify the source in disease and injury:

Referred pain

- *Shoulder:* from undersurface of diaphragm
- *Tip of scapula:* from gallbladder
- *Left chest:* from spleen
- *Umbilicus:* from appendix or pancreas
- *Groin/testes:* from ureter.

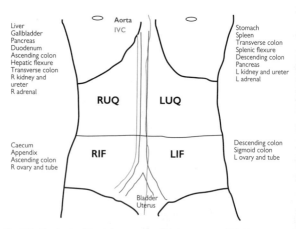

Fig. 14.1 Quadrants of the abdomen and underlying structures. This figure was published in *Sports Injury Assessment and Rehabilitation*, David C. Reid, p.716, figure 18.28, Copyright Elsevier (1991).

Table 14.1 Abdominal content

Solid organs	Hollow viscera
Liver	Stomach
Spleen	Small bowel
Pancreas	Large bowel
Kidneys	Gallbladder
Adrenals	Ureters
	Vasculature

Preparation and risk management

Reduce risks by ensuring:
- Appropriate protective equipment and adherence to rules
- Resting and using a staged return after injury and illness
- Relevant immunizations, especially if taking athletes abroad
- Especially when travelling observe good food hygiene and use clean water to avoid food poisoning/traveller's diarrhea.

Does an athlete require special protection or restriction of activities?
- *Previous liver laceration or trauma*: ↑ risk of further injury
- Congenital absence, loss of kidney, or testicle
- Bleeding disorders
- Sickle cell trait: ↑ risk of splenic infarction at moderate altitude
- Abdominal surgery: can usually return to training at 4 weeks, contact sports at 6–12 weeks or up to 6 months, depending on procedure
- *Glandular fever*: ✦ ↑ risk of splenic rupture.
  - Rest for duration of fever and return to contact sports only when back to full strength and FBC, LFTs, urinalysis and spleen size normal
  - The spleen normally takes up to 6–8 weeks to return to normal size and it is advisable to wait ~3 months before returning to contact sports unless an ultrasound can confirm normal size prior to this.

Know your athletes' Past medical history (PMHx)—ideally prior to any incidents. Underlying conditions may present with abdominal symptoms/signs:
- Diabetes mellitus
- Coeliac disease
- Inflammatory bowel disease
- Peptic ulcer disease
- Gallstones.

:⚙: Trauma

Mechanism of injury

Blunt

Compression and crushing forces from direct blows can damage solid organs and rupture hollow viscera leading to bleeding and peritonitis.

- Kicks, punches, head-butting (especially with helmet), stamping in a ruck in rugby, trampling by a horse in equestrian events
- Collapse of a maul in rugby, pile-on in American football
- *Missiles:* balls (baseball, cricket), pucks
- *Equipment:* bats, sticks, gymnastic apparatus
- Deceleration forces can tear mobile structures at their points of fixed attachment (spleen, liver, small bowel):
  - *Fall from a height:* equestrian events, gymnastics, diving
  - Crashes in motor sport.

Penetrating

- Not commonly seen in sport.
- Stab or slash wounds cause cutting or lacerating injury
- Gunshot wounds may cause additional damage through cavitation, tumbling, and fragmentation
- Penetrating spleen or liver injuries from fractured ribs are sometimes seen.

Assessment

▶▶In the acutely-injured athlete the aim is a rapid focused assessment in the field, while summoning on-site help and arranging emergency transfer.

- **A**irway (with C-spine immobilization) and **B**reathing must be secured as per the initial assessment described in 📖 pp.13–14)
- In the assessment of **C**irculation obvious sources of bleeding should be controlled with direct pressure to any bleeding point, and splinting of fractures
- If possible large-bore IV access should be established and analgesia administered as needed
- There is no role for IM morphine in an acutely injured athlete due to unpredictable absorption rates
- Opiates should only be administered by the IV route
- Signs of shock should be sought—repeatedly
- Presence of tachycardia, narrowed pulse pressure, hypotension after abdominal trauma mandate emergent transfer to an appropriate hospital with appropriate fluid resuscitation (see 📖 Chapter 2)
- Imaging via computed tomography (CT) or focused assessment with sonography for trauma (FAST) scanning in the emergency department with subsequent surgical intervention will be required if a sustained response is not achieved

- In the haemodynamically normal athlete findings suggestive of significant injury again necessitate transfer for further management
- ▶Blunt abdominal trauma may be associated with delayed onset of haemorrhage and/or peritonitis and repeated assessment and adequate advice to the athlete are important.

Specific injuries

Diaphragm

- Traumatic rupture is usually associated with significant blunt abdominal trauma and commonest on the left (right protected by liver)
- Herniation of abdominal contents into the thorax can cause collapse of the left lung and respiratory embarrassment
- Chest X-ray (CXR) is usually abnormal and surgical repair required
- Small tears may be missed initially and present delayed or when herniated bowel becomes ischaemic.

Spleen

- The normal spleen lies under the diaphragm against the posterior 9th–11th ribs
- A solid, firm organ about the size of the palm of the hand and rarely damaged by direct blunt trauma in sport, it may be vulnerable to deceleration or trauma from fractured ribs
- Splenic enlargement occurs in a number of conditions (glandular fever, lymphoma, leukaemia, etc.) and, in this state, injury is much more likely
- Injuries are often missed—a slow leak of blood may be initially symptom-free followed by dull left flank and left shoulder tip pain (Kehr's sign)
- Subcapsular haematoma can lead to delayed rupture
- Most splenic injuries can be managed conservatively with careful observation
- Splenectomy may be required for significant bleeding or injury.

Liver

- Direct blows can cause subcapsular haematoma, usually associated with significant pain and tenderness
- Lacerations are rarely seen in sport, but may result from deceleration in falls from a height and in motor sport.

Stomach

Injury is unusual, but may be produced by epigastric spearing, e.g. by a hockey stick. Acidic stomach contents cause early peritoneal irritation, and there may be bloody gastric aspirate and free air on X-ray.

Pancreas

- May rarely be injured by direct trauma causing compression against the vertebral column (cycle handlebars) or by deceleration
- Clues are epigastric tenderness, pain radiating to the back, or an ileus (distention, absent bowel sounds)
- Amylase may be ↑, CT/endoscopic retrograde cholecystic pancreatogram (ERCP) are often required.

Duodenum and small bowel

Air trapped between a closed pylorus and duodeno-jejunal junction at the time of blunt trauma can result in rupture of the duodenum. Retroperitoneal position means signs of injury are difficult to detect. Bloody gastric aspirate or retroperitoneal air on X-ray suggests the diagnosis.

- Proximal jejunum and distal ileum are vulnerable to deceleration forces which produce tearing near fixed points of attachment
- There may be an associated lumbar spine fracture
- Persistent pain and progressive abdominal signs develop due to peritonitis, but signs may be subtle initially.

Large bowel

Significant rupture from blunt trauma results in massive peritoneal contamination and is often associated with other injuries. Onset of peritonitis may be delayed with small, isolated tears.

Genito-urinary

- Sporting injury is the commonest cause of renal trauma
- The kidneys are relatively protected by the lower ribs, fat, and psoas muscles, but remain vulnerable to direct blows to the back/flank. which result in crushing between the 12th rib and lumbar spine
- Renal contusion causes flank pain which may radiate to the costovertebral junction or lower abdomen with gross haematuria ± renal colic (clots)
- There are usually external signs of injury and tenderness over the loin with rigidity of the anterior abdominal wall
- Immediately refer to hospital any athlete with gross haematuria or signs of shock for further investigation—usually contrast CT
- Approximately 95% of such injuries can be managed expectantly and hypovolaemic shock is almost always due to other injuries (which will also almost all be picked up by CT)
- By contrast, disruption of the renal pedicle, injuries to the ureter, and renal vessels are rare in sport
- They are seen with deceleration, rarely cause haematuria, and are serious and potentially life-threatening, presenting with severe shock and requiring prompt surgical intervention
- Therefore, do not discount significant renal injury just because there is no gross bleeding when the patient passes urine (PU)
- Microscopic haematuria is unlikely to be detected pitchside
- If there is access to a urine dipstix and the result is positive for blood then as long as the athletes observations are normal and there is not a concerning mechanism of injury (such as high speed road traffic accident (RTA)) then the athlete can be managed conservatively and referral to hospital is unlikely to be required unless his clinical condition changes
- A repeat urine dip should be carried out in a further 2 weeks to ensure the microscopic bleeding has resolved
- If still present then referral to urology will be required to look for other causes of haematuria.

Rectus abdominis injury

- Paired rectus abdominis muscles run vertically either side of the linea alba from 5th–7th costal cartilages to pubic bone.
  - They are segmented by fibrous intersections adherent to the muscle sheath which becomes continuous with the aponeuroses of the lateral muscles
  - Superior and inferior epigastric arteries enter the sheath and run along the posterior surface of the rectus muscles
- The muscles can be damaged by direct blows or strained. Strain injuries can be classified as:
  - Grade 1 mild—no effect on exercise ability. Pain usually after activity
  - Grade 2 moderate—pain at the time of injury with pain reproduced contracting the muscle
  - Grade 3 severe—pain at time, debilitating
- Return to sport will clearly depend on the grade of injury from 2–3 weeks for grade 1, 4–6 for grade 2 and up to 3 months for grade 3
- A rectus abdominis haematoma occurs due to rupture of one of the epigastric arteries—usually the inferior epigastric. This is due to stretching of the vessel
- Most haematomas form below the umbilicus and are tamponaded by the sheath.
- Presentation is with sudden pain and a well-localized immobile mass, which does not cross the midline or lateral muscle border, and is present on sitting and lying
- Marked tenderness and guarding may make differentiation from an intra-abdominal problem difficult and necessitate imaging
- Athletes who are in extreme pain or with signs of shock should be immediately referred to hospital as occasionally surgical evacuation may be needed and very rarely bleeding from the damaged vessels continues leading to shock if not recognized.

⚠ Significant muscle/SC haematoma after minimal trauma may indicate an underlying blood disorder, such as leukaemia or Idiopathic thrombocytopenic purpura (ITP). Athletes with repeated bruising out of proportion to the mechanism of injury should have the above conditions considered, especially when associated with recurrent nosebleeds or anaemia. A full blood count (FBC) and coagulation should be performed by the athlete's general practitioner.

Investigation of traumatic abdominal injury

- ▶Haemodynamic instability, which does not show a sustained response to crystalloid/blood, is an indication for surgical intervention, not imaging
- This will always be carried out from the nearest appropriate Emergency Department (ED) and transfer should not be delayed if the athlete's condition is unstable
- A number of investigations can be performed (see Table 14.2 for comparisons):
  - Increasingly CT scan is the preferred option due to increased speed of the equipment and ready availability
  - In the ED a FAST scan may easily be performed at the bedside and is highly specific though less sensitive than CT.

Table 14.2 Comparison of diagnostic peritoneal lavage (DPL), FAST, and CT for evaluation of abdominal trauma

	DPL	FAST	CT
Type of patient	Haemodynamically abnormal	Haemodynamically abnormal	Haemodynamically normal and co-operative, sedated, or anaesthetized
Look for	Blood, GI contents, bile	Fluid	Organ injury, fluid, pneumoperitoneum
Advantages	Quick, bedside, high sensitivity (96–100%)	Quick, bedside, non-invasive, repeatable, high specificity (up to 99%) for injuries requiring surgery, can be used for other body areas	Anatomical detail, quantifies haemorrhage, identifies on-going bleeding, good for retroperitoneum, sensitivity ~97%, specificity ~95%
Disadvantages	Invasive, risk of perforation, misses diaphragm or retroperitoneal injury	Low –ive predictive value, operator dependant, bowel gas/subcutaneous emphysema = distortion, misses clotted blood, diaphragm, bowel, some pancreatic injuries	Expensive, time-consuming, requires transfer, conventional scan may miss bowel, diaphragm and some pancreatic injuries, contrast and radiation exposure

:☼: Non-traumatic emergencies

Athletes may present with the full spectrum of abdominal and gastrointestinal (GI) complaints seen in the general population.

▶▶As for any acutely unwell athlete, assessment and management is guided by ABCDs with urgent transfer to hospital.

Acute cholecystitis

- Gallstone impaction in the biliary tree causes acute RUQ pain, which may radiate to back or shoulders
- There may be fever, sweating, nausea, and vomiting ± jaundice. Right upper quadrant (RUQ) tenderness/peritonism is maximal on inspiration (Murphy's sign)
- Rigors imply progression to cholangitis (infection)
- Admission to hospital will be required with IV fluids, anti-emetics, analgesia, and antibiotics the mainstay of treatment
- If cholecystectomy is required then this can be done either as an open procedure or laparascopically
- Return to sport will depend on the procedure and the sport performed, but may be as early as 2 weeks.

Acute liver failure

- Relevant causes in athletes include:
  - Exertional heatstroke
  - Paracetamol excess
  - Viral hepatitis, rarely as a side effect of anabolic steroids or creatine
- *Presentation:* jaundice, fever, nausea, vomiting, hepato(spleno)megaly, and/or complications such as hypoglycemia, bleeding, encephalopathy, sepsis, hepatorenal syndrome
- ▶Check and correct using blood glucose monitor (BM).

Appendicitis

- Commonest cause of acute abdomen in the UK, mainly in young adults and teenagers
- Presents with colicky peri-umbilical pain localizing to the right iliac fossa (RIF), anorexia, nausea, or diarrhoea
- There may be fever, flushed appearance, tachycardia, tenderness (rebound), and guarding in RIF maximal over McBurney's point with pain there on pressing in the left iliac fossa (LIF) (Rovsing's sign)
- Peritonitis, sepsis, and shock occur with perforation
- Return to play will again depend on whether there was associated perforation and the nature of the operation whether an open or laparoscopic procedure
- A graded return to activity starting with gentle exercise 2–4 weeks after operation should be expected in uncomplicated cases.

Inflammatory bowel disease

- Ulcerative colitis is commoner in ♀ and non-smokers
- Commoner than Crohn's and the commonest cause of prolonged bloody diarrhoea in the UK
- Suspect if 'infective gastroenteritis' fails to resolve
- Initial treatment is with fluid and electrolyte replacement. This has particular importance in athletes with a history of inflammatory bowel disease (IBD) and concomitant gastroenteritis/traveller's diarrhoea
- Acute complications include dehydration, haemorrhage, toxic dilatation, intestinal obstruction (Crohn's), perforation, and sepsis.

Indicators of a severe attack

- Abdominal pain
- >6 bloody stools, day, pus
- Systemically unwell
- Signs of hypoproteinaemia/anaemia
- Abdominal distention, tenderness, rebound
- Shock

Intestinal obstruction

- Presents with colicky abdominal pain, anorexia, nausea, vomiting (early if small bowel), abdominal distention (less if small bowel), constipation—not always absolute, 'tinkling' bowel sounds
- Fever and peritonism imply strangulation
- Commonly due to adhesions or herniae, more rarely tumour, ingested foreign body, gallstone ileus, intussusception, volvulus, or Crohn's
- Athletes in sports where intra-abdominal pressure is raised (e.g. weight-lifting) maybe more at risk of hernia formation including at unusual sites such as Spigelian (lateral border of rectus muscles, most often below the umbilicus, and difficult to palpate).

Paralytic ileus

This adynamic form of obstruction occurs more commonly in children with various causes including—gastroenteritis, hypokalaemia, narcotics.

Strangulated hernia

Athletes involved in heavy lifting are at risk of hernias and this may become strangulated. Always check the hernial orifices and femoral orifice for irreducible masses in patients with non-specific abdominal pain.

Pancreatitis

- Presents with severe epigastric pain, which may radiate to the back and is often better when leaning forward (pancreatic position)
- Often accompanied by vomiting
- Chief causes are gallstones and alcohol
- Drugs may be relevant in athletes and many have been implicated, both prescribed (sulphonamides, metronidazole, tetracyclines, sodium valproate, etc.) and those used for 'performance enhancement', e.g. steroids or diuretics in sports with weight limits or where low body weight is advantageous, such as boxing and gymnastics
- Third spacing of fluid can be substantial leading to shock

- Necrosis and bleeding may produce periumbilical (Cullen's sign) or flank discolouration (Grey Turner's sign).

Upper gastrointestinal bleed

- Presents with haematemesis and/or melaena
- Fit athletes can remain haemodynamically normal despite significant blood loss, i.e. postural dizziness or hypotension may be an early sign of incipient collapse
- Peptic ulcer disease and oesophagitis/gastritis account for 80%
- Non-steroidal anti-inflammatory drug (NSAID) use may be associated
- Rarer causes:
  - Mallory–Weiss tear (commonly after excess alcohol)
  - Crohn's
  - Meckel's diverticulum (fresher per rectum (pr) blood, ♂>♀)
  - Vascular malformations
  - Malignancy
  - Coagulopathy/platelet disorder.

ⓘ Minor injuries and conditions

Stitch
- Sharp pain (usually around right lower ribs)
- Commonly seen in less fit individuals and when exercising too soon after eating
- Actual aetiology is unknown, but various conditions have been proposed, such as the diaphragm being pulled when the solid organs stretch as you exercise
- Can 'run through' by leaning over to that side, pressing with fingers or stretching up the arm on the affected side, breathing out through pursed lips. May need to lie with arms above head/legs bent
- Specific breathing exercises may help to prevent it occurring, such as timing of respiration relating to running stride.

Winding
- A blow to the abdomen when muscles are relaxed can lead to the athlete feeling unable to breathe freely (diaphragmatic spasm). This can therefore cause great distress
- Check **A**irway and **B**reathing, loosen clothing, encourage the athlete to relax, and sit leaning forward over flexed knees
- Normal breathing usually returns quickly
- Ensure there is no serious underlying injury by monitoring pulse and BP
- Symptoms should settle quickly, but if they persist or worsen then intra-abdominal injury should be considered and referral to hospital made.

Skin wounds
- Irrigate and cover with an occlusive, non-adherent dressing
- Any suggestion that depth extends to muscle or beyond, apply pressure if necessary and transfer to hospital.

Skin irritation
- Torso skin may be affected by contact dermatitis, e.g. from nickel in clothing/equipment or from plants—poison ivy, primula, etc.
- Treatment is with cold compresses, steroid cream, and avoidance of irritants.
- Intertrigo is an irritant dermatitis in skin folds (submammary, groin) due to the combination of sweat and friction
- Treatment is as before, plus attention to secondary fungal or bacterial infection.

Gastrointestinal complaints
- Heartburn, nausea, vomiting, and loss of appetite are all common ♀ > ♂ particularly with intense activity and in less experienced athletes
- Importance lies in excluding serious underlying causes (peptic ulcer disease, ischaemic heart disease (IHD)), symptoms may respond to dietary and/or activity modification
- Faecal occult blood loss is very common in endurance athletes

- Again, importance lies in excluding underlying causes. Proper hydration and prophylactic H_2 blocker may help.
- Nausea, stomach cramps, and diarrhoea may be seen with creatine use
- *Traveller's diarrhoea* (nausea, watery diarrhoea, cramps) is most often due to *E. coli* and lasts 3–5 days
- Oral fluid and electrolyte rehydration is usually sufficient. Loperamide (not with fever or dysentery) or bismuth may help, antibiotics (co-trimoxazole) are reserved for protracted illness.

Athletic pseudonephritis

- Abnormal urinalysis is common after strenuous aerobic activity particularly in long-distance runners
- Red blood cell count (RBC), white blood cell count (WBC), haemoglobin (Hb), myoglobin, protein, and casts may all be seen and on occasion gross haematuria
- The condition is benign, usually causes at most mild discomfort and settles with rest from strenuous activity for 24–48 h
- Persistent symptoms warrant investigation.

Pelvic trauma

Introduction

- Pelvic trauma is common in the world of sport. It is a spectrum ranging from a simple strain to a devastating, life-threatening pelvic ring fracture
- Despite being common it can be notoriously difficult to diagnose accurately with many injuries presenting in a similar fashion
- It also has to be remembered that there are many non-muscular structures in this area that may be the cause of pain and pain is often referred to the knee
- An accurate diagnosis is key to allowing appropriate treatment and rehabilitation.

Anatomy

- The hip and pelvis are two distinct, but interrelated parts of the human body:
  - The bony pelvis connects the trunk and legs, supporting the trunk and containing intestine, urinary bladder, and the internal sex organs
  - The bony pelvis comprises 3 bones on either side—the ilium, ischium, and pubis
- Anteriorly the pubic bones are united by a cartilaginous joint known as the pubic symphisis
- Posteriorly the bony sacrum connects with both ilia at the sacroiliac joints and its upper portion provides connection with the vertebral column
- The acetabulum is the concave surface of the pelvis formed by the fusion of the 3 pelvic bones
- It meets with the head of the femur and together they form the hip joint
- The hip joint is a ball and socket joint capable of an extensive range of movement (see Table 15.1).

Table 15.1 Muscles of the hip

Movement	Muscle
Flexion	Sartorius, rectus femoris, iliopsoas (iliacus and psoas)
Extension	Gluteus maximus, hamstrings
Adduction	Gracilis, pectineus, adductor longus, adductor brevis, adductor magnus
Abduction	Gluteus medius, gluteus minimus, tensor fascia lata
External rotation	Gluteus minimus, piriformis, obturator internus, quadratus femoris
Internal rotation	Gluteus medius, adductor magnus, semimebranosus, semitendinosus

Assessment

History

- At the pitchside the most important part of the initial assessment is to secure the airway, breathing, and circulation (ABC)
- The pelvis is included as part of the circulation assessment as a significant volume of blood that can be lost due to a fracture in this area
- Obtain details of the mechanism of injury
- This may come from direct observation of the injury at the pitchside, from the athlete or team-mates
- A history of allergy, medications, past medical history, last eaten, events preceding (AMPLE) history is appropriate in initial assessment:
  - Injury mechanism—was the trauma direct, e.g. fall from horse, or indirect, e.g. sprinting or jumping? Was the trauma a high or low impact/velocity, e.g. motor vehicle crash at speed? Was there any associated twisting/rotational component either of the back or of the hip (especially with the foot planted)?
  - Mobility—has the athlete been able to weight-bear since, i.e. could he carry on and continue to compete or has he not been able to stand since? Is the pain localized to one specific area, e.g. muscle insertion? Is the pain there constantly or only when actively moving?
  - Were there any preceding problems that make the clinical assessment more difficult, e.g. is there a history of osteitis pubis, previous surgery, or injuries to the pelvis, groin, hip, or lower back?
- From the AMPLE history make a plan about how best to analgese the athlete, i.e. contra-indications to non-steroid anti-inflammatory drugs (NSAIDs)
- ♀ *Last menstrual period*: worth noting in females of child-bearing age as conditions such as ectopic pregnancy may be missed or initially attributed to problems such as groin strain:
  - X-rays of the pelvis may need to be taken in hospital as part of the initial 'primary' assessment in a significant injury
  - Being aware of the pregnancy status can prove helpful in determining specific films taken and minimizing radiation doses.

Examination

Look

- For any swelling, bruising, or deformity
- Previous scars
- Observe gait if the athlete is able to walk
- Do not force them to their feet until you are have made a full assessment of their active then passive movements to ensure that no further harm will result from them weight-bearing.

Feel

- For any tenderness, warmth, crepitations, etc.
- Check pulses and assess the neurovascular status of the lower limbs.

Move

- Assess the active range of movement before the passive
- Perform any specific tests appropriate for the affected area.

☼ Fractures and dislocations

Fractures

Pelvic ring fractures
- Fractures to the pelvis are a result of high energy blunt trauma
- They are associated with a high morbidity and mortality secondary to complications from the fracture itself and associated injuries
- As with all major injuries the ABCD assessment must be followed and associated cervical spine injury considered
- Pelvic fractures are commonly seen in the equestrian, motorsport, and cycling environments
- Pelvic fractures occur as a result of one of three loading forces, lateral compression, anterior posterior (AP) compression (open book), and vertical shear (Table 15.2).

Table 15.2 Loading forces causing pelvic fractures

Force	Example of force
Lateral compression	Side impact in motor vehicle accident
AP compression	Head on collision in vehicle accident
Vertical shear	Fall from height

Treatment
- Resuscitate ABCD (📖 Chapter 2)
- Obtain IV access as soon as possible. Give analgesia with morphine and start IV fluids if available
- ⚠ Do not attempt to 'spring' the pelvis as it is unreliable and may cause further damage
- Use pelvic splint if available to tamponade and stop bleeding. A number of these are commercially available, but a sheet tied around the pelvis may be a useful temporizing measure
- Continue to monitor pulse and blood pressure (BP)
- Transfer urgently to definitive centre.

Complications
- Haemorrhage is the most serious immediate complication of pelvic fracture
- Massive retroperitoneal haemorrhage may occur from bony fragments and lacerated blood vessels
- The retroperitoneal space can hold up to 4 L of blood before tamponade occurs
- Continued bleeding may therefore result in shock
- Associated injuries are extremely common owing to the huge forces involved. The most common are:
  - Head injury
  - Long bone fracture
  - Nerve injury (sacral plexus, sciatic)

- Thoracic injury
- Urethra
- Bladder
- Intra-abdominal solid and hollow viscus organs
- Diaphragm.

Sacral fractures

- May occur in isolation or as part of a pelvic fracture with or without sacro-iliac joint disruption. 30% present late, and delay in presentation is associated with an increased incidence of chronic pain and neurological dysfunction
- Again equestrian sports are particularly linked to this type of injury
- Fractures may be transverse or vertical, and due to the possibility of neurological involvement around the sacral foramina it is vital that a full neurological assessment is made
- Note the athlete may still be able to mobilize after the injury with the only finding being tenderness elicited by palpating the sacrum
- Return to sport will usually be a minimum of 6–8 weeks, but may be longer depending on the sport.

Initial management

- In the initial stages of assessment it may be very difficult to distinguish the athlete suffering from an uncomplicated sacral fracture from someone suffering a complicated pelvic injury and so initial treatment as per ABCD should be carried out
- Unless the athlete is mobile, transfer to hospital is likely to be required and imaging initially with plain film X-rays will be necessary
- Further imaging with computed tomography (CT) may be required along with magnetic resonance imaging (MRI) should there be any evidence of neurological involvement.

Avulsion fractures

- These fractures are most commonly seen in the adolescent age group
- They are due to the sudden forceful contraction of a muscle pulling a piece of the bone off
- There are 3 main sites involved (Table 15.3).

Table 15.3 Location of avulsion fracture

Site	Muscle	Action
Anterior superior iliac spine (ASIS)	Sartorius	Jumping
Anterior inferior iliac spine (AIIS)	Rectus femoris	Kicking, e.g. football
Ischial tuberosity	Hamstrings	Sprinting, hurdling

- Athletes may describe a sudden pop followed by pain in the hip or groin
- Tenderness is elicited by palpating the affected site and bruising may be noted
- Distinction between injuries with associated avulsion fractures and those without, i.e. musculotendinous strains may be very difficult

- If the history is suggestive and there is specific insertion tenderness then X-rays should be obtained
- Generally, these injuries will settle with rest and conservative management, but sometimes they may not heal or the fragment may be too large
- Referral to orthopaedic services is recommended for follow-up as soon as a bony avulsion has been identified to allow a decision regarding operative treatment to be made
- In general, if the X-ray demonstrates more than 2 cm displacement of the bony fragment from the pelvis then operative management will be preferred to allow a quicker return to play.

Stress fractures
- Stress fractures are the result of overuse injuries
- Fatigued muscles transfer the stress to the bone causing a fracture
- In the pelvic region they are most commonly seen in either the pubic rami or neck of femur
- Runners, especially long distance, are the group most likely to be affected
- Military trainees are also a high risk group
- Females suffer more than males: this is probably related to hormone-induced osteoporosis
- Palpation of the ramus will prove tender if a fracture is present, but neck of femur fractures are more difficult to diagnose
- In femoral neck stress fractures a high degree of suspicion is required in those most at risk
- Patients will complain of a pain in the anterior groin that worsens with activity and resolves with rest
- It may then progress to being constant
- Pain may radiate to the knee and may be described as a deep-seated ache
- X-rays should be undertaken, but often the fracture is not visible. CT or MRI may be needed to allow diagnosis
- Operative fixation will be required in the vast majority of cases and urgent orthopaedic referral will be required
- Complications include avascular necrosis and non-union (if conservative management is used.)

Acetabular fractures
- Rarely occur in isolation as they too are a result of high energy forces
- They are commonly associated with pelvic ring fractures and hip dislocations
- Complications, associated injuries, and assessment are the same as for pelvic ring fractures.

Dislocation of the hip
- Dislocations of the hip can be posterior, anterior, or central
- Dislocation of the hip requires a significant force and other injuries are common
- Posterior dislocations account for approx 90% of hip dislocations in sports

- They occur when great force strikes the flexed knee with the hip flexed, adducted, and internally rotated
- They are most commonly seen in contact sports like American football and rugby, where players are tackled and land with other players piling on top of them. They have also been documented in motor sports, skiing, and snowboarding.

Examination
In a posterior dislocation typically the leg is shortened, internally rotated, with flexion and adduction at the hip.

Initial management
- Resuscitate per ABCD
- Obtain IV access and give analgesia (with opiate if possible)
- Assess neurovascular status of the affected limb. The sciatic nerve and its common peroneal branch are most commonly involved in posterior dislocations:
  - Look for foot drop, and decreased power and sensation
  - Ensure you assess the knee joint as well for associated fractures
- Arrange urgent transfer to hospital
- There is a significant increase in long term hip joint damage if the hip is not reduced within 6 h
- There are reports of this being managed at the pitchside in the first few minutes after dislocation before muscle spasm intervenes
- This can only be advised if the operator has experience in the techniques used to achieve this, and it would be expected that this procedure is usually carried out in a hospital environment.

Return to play
- Imaging will usually be carried out at 6 weeks to ensure no signs of avascular necrosis
- Gentle jogging may then be undertaken with a full return to sport between 4–6 months post-injury.

① **Soft tissue injuries**

Soft tissue injuries are common in athletes. The incidence of these may be reduced by an adequate warm up and stretching programme prior to the activity. Evidence for this, however, is still controversial.

Strains

Strains occur when the muscle fibres tear as a result of overstretching. They can be graded into three severities, but it can be difficult to grade them accurately (Table 15.4).

Table 15.4 Grades of strain

Grade	Description
I (mild)	Stretching or minor tearing of a ligament or muscle
II (moderate)	Ligament or muscle partially torn, but still intact
III (severe)	Ligament or muscle is completely torn and joint is unstable

Adductor strain

- Occur where there is a violent external rotation with the leg in a widely abducted position
- Changing direction suddenly in sports such as tennis, basketball, and tackles in football can all be responsible
- Injuries are often acute on chronic
- Many perceive this to be an overuse injury
- A number of factors may contribute to development of an adductor strain including imbalances between the strength of the adductors and the gluteal muscles
- Acute injuries will present with the athlete often describing a sudden, sharp, ripping pain in the affected groin
- There may be previous experience of niggling groin pain in this area
- They may be swelling and tenderness over the origin of the adductor and there will be pain on resisted adduction
- Initial treatment of the acute injury involves withdrawal from play, rest, and ice
- Compression bandages may be symptomatically helpful
- Mainstay of treatment of these injuries is identifying those with chronic strains and rehabilitating them before a superimposed acute injury occurs
- Once identified, strengthening the adductors, and core exercises is crucial in these cases prior to return to full activity
- Length of time away from play is dependent on a number of factors, such as the grade of strain, and the response to a controlled, supervised rehabilitation programme
- MRI or ultrasound (US) scanning may be very useful in determining the extent of the injury and assessing for other differential diagnoses
- Chronic injuries may take up to 6 months to fully settle.

Hip flexor strain

- The hip flexors are the rectus femoris (which is also involved in knee extension) iliacus and psoas
- Any or all three muscles may be affected though iliopsoas is most commonly affected
- Hip flexor strains tend to occur either as a result of an explosive movement such as a burst of speed when running or when striking an object with your foot—such as a ball
- Pain is present over the anterior upper thigh and is associated with movements involving the flexors
- This can be assessed by asking the athlete to bring his knee towards his chest—the pain may be reproduced on resisted extension of the hip
- It may be confused with an adductor strain, but can be differentiated by the absence of pain with lateral movements
- Treatment is usually symptomatic with rest and ice progressing to ultrasound and massage under the direction of the physiotherapists
- Return to play will again depend on the grade of strain but may take up to 6 weeks.

Hamstring strain

- Account for approximately 1/3 of all sports-related lower limb injuries, and are recurrent in about 1/3
- Injuries tend to occur in sports such as football that require explosive extension of the knee, as when sprinting
- Symptoms may be insidious, but are more likely to be dramatic with the athlete pulling up 4 or 5 strides into a sprint
- An audible pop may be heard. There will be point tenderness over the injured muscle and possibly extending to the ischial tuberosity
- A palpable defect may be present and muscle spasm evident
- MRI will define the extent of the injury as well as excluding associated avulsion fracture of the ischium
- Plain films may be useful if there is a question of associated fracture and MRI is unavailable
- Initial treatment involves withdrawal from play, ice, and compressive bandages. Analgesia and the use crutches is recommended until able to mobilize without pain
- A graded return to full activities will be required using a supervised rehabilitation programme. As a rough guide:
  - Grade 1 strains—2–3 weeks
  - Grade 2 strains—3–6 weeks
  - Grade 3 strains—6–8 weeks

! **Other causes of acute pelvic pain**

Slipped upper femoral epiphysis

- Seen in the 10–17-years age group, ♂>♀(3:1). Occurs in left leg more than right
- May present as sudden onset groin pain following trauma, or insidiously over weeks as gradually increasing groin pain or worsening limp
- Pain may be felt in the groin, medial thigh, or the knee. Up to 40% of patients will develop bilateral involvement
- The patient may hold their hip in external rotation, with pain reproducible on passive internal rotation
- Both AP and 'frog leg' views of the pelvis should be taken
- Operative fixation will be required so urgent orthopaedic review is necessary
- Prophylactic fixation of the contralateral limb remains controversial
- Supported weight bearing using crutches will usually be required for up to 8 weeks post-surgery with a return to play not advocated by some until the physis has closed.

Ectopic pregnancy

For any female of child-bearing age who presents with acute pelvic pain this must be kept in mind. Occurs in approximately 1% of pregnancies with 95% of ectopic pregnancies occurring in the fallopian tubes. Symptoms usually occur between weeks 4 and 10 of the pregnancy.

Symptoms may include:
- Unilateral groin pain
- Vaginal bleeding
- Postural hypotension
- Shock with tachycardia and decreased BP
- Shoulder tip pain.

Treatment will depend on the initial presentation, but if the patient is unstable then immediate surgery is warranted. Even if the patient has normal observations then bear in mind that deterioration can occur quickly and catastrophically if rupture occurs.
- Manage the patient by addressing the ABCs
- Cannulate and start IV fluid, as well as opiate for the pain
- Immediately transfer to the nearest Emergency Department (ED).

Return to sport is unlikely to be on the athletes mind, but will vary depending on the extent of the surgery required.

Testicular torsion

- Is a true urological emergency and can present with groin pain. It is most common in the men <30-years-old with most between the ages of 12 and 18 years
- The majority of patients will usually complain of acute onset of unilateral scrotal pain
- Torsion results in disruption of the blood supply to the teste and the teste itself will become non-viable if the torsion is not reversed. A success rate approaching 100% for retaining viability of the teste occurs if the procedure is done within 6 h of the onset of symptoms.

Symptoms
- Unilateral pain usually acute onset
- Lower abdominal pain
- Scrotal swelling
- Vomiting.

Signs
- *Swollen scrotum:* may be warm and red
- Markedly tender to palpation
- Teste lying horizontal (bell-clapper)
- Loss of cremasteric reflex on the affected side (not seen in epidiymitis)
- High temperature is unusual.

Diagnostic tests are usually not required as this is a clinical diagnosis.
  Blood tests have little value, but ultrasound may be useful as long as it does not delay the surgical procedure.

Treatment
Administer analgesia and immediately refer to the nearest ED—ideally one with on-site urology cover.
  Return to play can usually be around a month post-fixation.

Sports hernia (Gilmore's groin)
Commonly associated with kicking sports, such as football, rugby, and American football. It is caused by weakening of the posterior inguinal wall.
- Patients will complain of a gradual onset of deep groin pain
- The pain will increase with manoeuvres, which increase intra-abdominal pressure and may radiate to the testicles
- On examination there will be no palpable hernia as it is only the posterior abdominal wall that is involved
- Diagnosis is difficult and often by exclusion
- Patients should be referred for surgical assessment on an outpatient basis.

Osteitis pubis
- Is inflammation at the pubic symphysis caused by repetitive contraction of the muscles that attach to the pubic bones and pubic symphysis
- Pain has a gradual onset and tenderness is elicited when palpating the pubic symphysis
- It is most commonly seen in footballers and long distance runners though can be seen in dancers, ice skaters, and weight lifters
- It is more prevalent in ♂ aged 30–50 years
- It is not commonly encountered in the paediatric population.

Bursitis

Iliopsoas bursitis

- Is commonly associated with iliopsoas tendonitis due to their close proximity
- Together they are known as the iliopsoas syndrome
- Patients will describe anterior thigh pain and sometimes a snapping sensation in the hip
- There may be a palpable mass owing to the increasing size of the bursa.

Trochanteric bursitis

The trochanteric bursa has a superficial and deep component. Patients will normally describe lateral thigh pain. Pain can be reproduced by hip adduction (superficial) or resisted active abduction (deep).

Apophysitis

- An apophysis is a growth plate that provides a point for a muscle to attach to
- If the muscle attached is excessively tight it can put increased tension on the apophysis, which results in inflammation and apophysitis
- There are several at the pelvis that can be affected
- It most commonly affects adolescents who participate in running, dancing, and football
- They will complain of pain in the area of the associated apophysis, but it may be more diffuse and will worsen with activity
- X-rays are important to exclude avulsion fractures.

Upper limb injury

Introduction

Limb injuries, whilst unlikely to cause mortality, are the biggest cause of morbidity faced by athletes.

Upper limb sporting injuries are a common presentation to emergency departments. One of the most common mechanisms of injury occurs as a result of falling onto an outstretched hand (FOOSH) as a reflex reaction to a fall. Direct blows to the upper limb are also a common mechanism of injury, as are injuries secondary to ball-games resulting in hyperextension to the wrist.

Often injuries occur in individual sports in a manner that is predictable in both the mechanism of injury and presentation.

① Clavicular injuries

Assessment

- As with all orthopaedic trauma, assessment begins with 'look, feel, move' before assessment of distal neurovascular deficit
- There will be tenderness over the fracture site, and there may be obvious deformity and swelling at the fracture site acutely
- The patient will usually support the injured limb by holding the forearm
- Most clavicular injuries will severely limit movement at the gleno-humeral joint
- Acromio-clavicular injuries will cause pain on adduction of the arm across the chest with the elbow flexed.

Claviclular fractures

- Most clavicular injuries occur as a result of direct force to the shoulder, either as a direct fall or blow
- Clavicular injuries may also occur as a result of a FOOSH
- The commonest site of fracture is at the junction of the middle and outer thirds
- Middle third fractures are also common. Fractures of the outer third are less common and those of the medial third rarer still
- Adolescents and young adults will often fracture in a 'greenstick' pattern
- No manipulation or reduction of clavicle fractures is required acutely
- Approximately 3% of clavicle fractures will be associated with a pneumothorax so assessment of the chest is mandatory.

Acromio-clavicular injury

These often occur after a fall onto the shoulder. They are graded radio-logically, although deformity at the acromio-clavicular (AC) joint may be noted pitchside, with the distal tip of the clavicle sitting superiorly to the acromion.

Sterno-clavicular injury

- These are relatively rare and result from a blow to the front of the shoulder resulting in the clavicle 'popping' out anteriorly
- Asymmetry, swelling, and local tenderness of the medial end of the clavicle is noted compared with the other side
- △ Rarely the dislocation occurs posteriorly and can cause compressive symptoms on the mediastinal structures
- This will require surgical decompression with elevation of the dislocated clavicle
- CT is usually required to confirm this diagnosis as it is commonly not picked up on plain imaging.

Treatment

- Acute treatment entails supporting the arm in a broad arm or polysling, usually with the elbow at 90° of flexion. However, do not force the arm into this position—the patient is likely to present in their own 'position of comfort'
- Definitive treatment for clavicle fractures can either be conservative with operative fixation a consideration in displaced fractures
- Return to play is variable depending on factors such as the age of the athlete the displacement of the fracture fragments and the sport
- An adult returning to contact sports is likely to require up to 3 months or so of rehabilitation.

⚠ Shoulder injuries

Dislocations

The gleno-humeral joint may disclocate anteriorly, posteriorly, or inferi-orly. The vast majority of dislocations are anterior.

Anterior dislocation

- These usually occur from a FOOSH when the shoulder is externally rotated or where the trunk rotates internally after a FOOSH
- The patient will be in immediate pain and will support the upper limb with the opposite hand, at the elbow, or forearm
- The shoulder will often look 'squared off' in less muscular subjects
- Palpation under the acromion will reveal a palpable gap
- If the axillary nerve is damaged then there may be paraesthesia in a 'badge' distribution over the deltoid.

Treatment

- Reduction should not be carried out pitchside unless
  - This is a recurrent injury that the sportsman has had before or
  - There is neurovascular compromise or
  - There will be a significant delay to hospital assessment
- The arm should be supported in a broad arm sling in a position of comfort to the patient.

Methods of reduction

- Analgesia will be required—Entonox® is ideal
- There are numerous methods of reduction of anterior dislocations, most of which involve a degree of abduction and external rotation of the shoulder
- All 3 techniques should be performed gently and gradually
  - Lie the athlete supine—support the affected arm and gently lift the arm in an upwards direction trying to achieve 90° flexion at the shoulder. If you continue to support the arm and gently pull skywards the athletes body weight will act as traction and the dislocation can reduce
  - Lie the athlete semi-recumbent—extend the elbow and apply gentle traction to pull the arm in a downwards direction. The operator should lean backwards whilst holding the athletes arm. No other force is required
  - Lie the athlete prone—with their arm hanging over the side of the treatment table. Ask them to hold onto a weight such as a heavy water bottle. Gravity will allow the dislocation to reduce
- A balance needs to be struck as to where and when to reduce
- There is always the possibility of an associated fracture and also the potential of medico-legal issues if this is found on imaging carried out in hospital after a pitchside reduction
- In athletes with significant swelling or any doubt as to the diagnosis then splint the arm in a sling and transfer for imaging.

Posterior dislocation
- The mechanism of injury is usually a fall onto an internally rotated hand or a direct blow to the front of the shoulder
- Classically, this occurs as a result of either a seizure or electric shock where the shoulder is forced into hyper internal rotation
- Clinically, there is usually no deformity
- The athlete will have pain on active and passive movement out of proportion to the clinical findings
- Administer analgesia, apply sling, and refer to hospital.

Inferior dislocation (luxio erecta)
- This injury is very rare (approximately 0.5% of shoulder dislocations)
- Usually seen in high impact motorsport accidents and occasionally in falls from height, such as in gymnastics
- The arm is usually fully abducted with the elbow held flexed and resting on or above the head
- Administer analgesia and refer to hospital.

Shoulder fractures
These can mimic dislocations with the patient presenting holding the injured arm supported with the other hand.

Neck of humerus fractures
These are relatively uncommon injuries in sport
- Commoner in the young and the elderly
- Usually the result of a FOOSH with or without a further load landing on top of the limb, i.e. another athlete
- The normal contour of the shoulder is unlikely to be lost, thus helping to distinguish it from an anterior dislocation
- X-ray will allow distinction of the type of injury and whether it involves the surgical or anatomical necks
- Fractures of the surgical neck may involve the brachial plexus, notably the axillary nerve and this should be looked for with paraesthesia in a badge distribution overlying the deltoid
- Administer analgesia, apply sling, and transfer to hospital
- Definitive treatment may be conservative or operative, but early rehabilitation is key in assisting a return to sport with contact sport usually taking about 3 months.

Scapula fracture
- Usually the result of a direct blow to the posterior chest wall
- Typically, affects the blade of the scapula with obvious bruising and swelling found on assessment
- Complications are related to the associated injuries that are sustained at the same time such as pneumothorax, haemothorax, and rib fractures
- A full ABC assessment must be carried out
- The vast majority of scapula fractures are treated conservatively with splinting using a sling, which can be fully discarded by about 6 weeks.

Shaft of humerus fractures
- These may result from a direct blow to the side of the arm or a FOOSH
- The diagnosis is rarely in doubt, with localized tenderness, swelling +/− bruising
- Complications include associated vascular injuries and radial nerve palsy resulting in wrist drop
- Check distal pulses and neurology
- Administer analgesia, provide a sling or collar and cuff, and refer to hospital
- Definitive treatment is usually conservative.

Rotator cuff injuries

The rotator cuff muscles serve to stabilize the glenohumeral joint.
- Supraspinatus initiates abduction
- Infraspinatus and teres minor are responsible for external rotation
- Subscapularis provides internal rotation.

Rotator cuff injuries are diagnoses of exclusion in terms of pitchside assessment. They are almost impossible to diagnose pitchside or indeed acutely as the hallmark of these injuries is weakness in function and pain. Since pain will limit the ability to move, these are most commonly diagnosed on MRI, US, or at subsequent examination once the acute pain has settled.

⚠ Elbow injuries

Dislocation

- Dislocated elbow may occur in isolation or with associated fracture. It may be closed or compound
- Clinical appearances will show a loss of the normal anatomical triangle formed between the olecranon and the medial and lateral epicondyles on either side
- A visible deformity will be present. There is usually considerable soft tissue swelling
- An immediate check must be made for the presence or loss of brachial and distal pulses, as well as the median and ulnar nerves, which can also be injured
- If there are absent pulses and no immediate nearby ED facility then consideration should be given to reducing the dislocation
- Most dislocations occur in a postero-lateral direction and reduction is usually achieved using 2 operators
  - The first operator stabilizes the upper arm with the elbow flexed
  - With a second person applying traction distally, the first operator uses their thumbs to push the olecranon in a distal direction
  - This should allow the dislocation to reduce and the normal 'triangle' appearance of the elbow to be restored
  - A check should be made of the neurovascular status and the patient immediately referred to hospital for imaging and definitive treatment.

Fractures

Supracondylar fractures

- These usually are as a result of a FOOSH and are commonest in childhood. They can cause vascular compromise by impinging on the brachial artery and neurological compromise by impinging on the ulnar nerve
- There will be significant swelling and tenderness but the triangular anatomical relationship between the olecranon and epicondyles will be intact
- Treatment involves analgesia, applying a sling and referral to hospital
- Operative management will be dictated by the age of the patient, the degree of angulation and displacement, as well as neurovascular status.

Radial head/neck fractures

- Usually caused by FOOSH
- Occasionally caused by direct blow to elbow
- Patient usually unable to fully extend and supinate elbow
- There will usually be point tenderness over the radial head or neck as well as a haemarthosis of the elbow joint
- Plain imaging is required and treatment is usually conservative in a sling, or collar and cuff.

Olecranon fracture

- The olecranon tends to fracture as the result of landing on the point of the elbow
- Localized bruising, tenderness, and swelling result
- Management depends on the displacement of the olecranon fragment caused by the pull of triceps with displaced fractures requiring operative fixation
- Administer analgesia, apply sling, and refer to hospital.

ⓘ **Forearm injuries**

Fractures

Isolated ulnar shaft fracture

- A direct blow to the forearm or a fall against a hard surface may result in an isolated fracture to the ulna
- This may also be seen in sports where 'defensive' injuries occur as a result of bringing the hands and forearms upwards to protect the face
- Localized tenderness and swelling may be apparent
- It is vital to check for the presence of an associated radial dislocation as these injuries can occur together
- Imaging will be required of the entire forearm in a suspected ulnar shaft fracture
- For this reason administer analgesia, apply sling, and refer to hospital
- Undisplaced fractures may be treated in a cast with displaced fractures requiring operative fixation.

Isolated radial shaft fracture

- Unusual injury to have an isolated fracture to the proximal 2/3rds of the radius
- Usually the result of a fall or direct blow
- Always assess and X-ray for associated dislocations
- Non operative treatment is rare.

Fractures to both radial and ulna shafts

- Usually the result of significant force
- Highly unstable as no ability for either bone to be splinted by the other
- Clinically apparent due to pain, swelling +/- deformity
- Assessment of neurovascular status is mandatory
- Internal fixation is almost always required.

Dislocations

Monteggia fracture dislocation

- Fractured shaft of ulna
- Dislocation of the radial head.

The elbow and wrist joints must be examined closely in any suspected forearm fracture in order to look for an associated dislocation of the radial head in an ulnar shaft fracture. X-ray will reveal both problems with operative fixation required to reduce the dislocation.

Galeazzi fracture dislocation

- Fractured shaft of radius between middle and distal thirds
- Dislocation of the distal radio-ulnar joint (wrist joint).

Mechanism is usually direct blows to the forearm or a fall. X-ray is again required to confirm the extent of the injuries and operative fixation is required.

⚠ Wrist injuries

Fractures

Distal radius and ulnar fractures

- These injuries are usually caused by a FOOSH or a hyperextension injury, e.g. being struck by a ball
- Distal radius fractures are the most common of the radius fractures
- They can occur in isolation or in conjunction with an ulnar fracture
- The majority of displaced fractures displace dorsally, resulting in a 'dinner fork' appearance
- Assessment of the median nerve is required, as well as palpation of the distal pulses
- These injuries may require manipulation, open reduction, and internal fixation or conservative management
- Any clinically obvious deformity will invariably mean that the patient will require manipulation of the fracture so splint, analgese, and refer to hospital
- Depending on the type of fracture it may be possible to return to sport relatively quickly wearing a custom fit splint in the case of an undisplaced radial styloid fracture for example. More commonly, it will take about 6 weeks.

Colle's fracture

Fracture of the radius within 2.5cm of the wrist joint with dorsal angulation. Classically-associated with an ulnar styloid fracture and causes a 'dinner-fork' type deformity.

Smith's fracture

Fracture of the radius with volar angulation. Usually as a result of falling onto a flexed wrist.

Barton's fracture

Unstable intra-articular fracture of the volar aspect of the distal radius extending into the wrist joint.

Scaphoid fractures

- Usually caused by a FOOSH, causing swelling and tenderness in the anatomical snuffbox and tenderness on axial loading of the thumb or index finger
- Also assess for tenderness of the volar aspect of the scaphoid tubercle
- Due to the intricate blood supply, avasular necrosis can occur and so treatment of the 'clinical' diagnosis with splintage or casting is mandatory even in the presence of normal X-rays
- MRI if available will provide a definitive diagnosis. If unavailable immediately then follow up is required in 10–14 days after injury even in the presence of a normal X-ray
- Return to sport is usually in the order of 6–12 weeks.

Dislocation

Lunate dislocation

- Usually the result of FOOSH
- Whilst there will be pain and swelling, the symptoms will usually be out of keeping with the signs
- Paraesthesia in the median nerve distribution may be apparent and is a pointer to the diagnosis
- X-ray is required to confirm although the appearance is only truly appreciated on the lateral view
- Reduction is required so administer analgesia and refer.

Peri-lunate dislocation

- Uncommon in sport
- The result of high velocity forces
- Usually associated with significant swelling, but occasionally this is not the case
- There is significant soft tissue disruption including ligamentous rupture. The lunate maintains its alignment with the radius (in comparison with a lunate dislocation), whilst the capitate is displaced dorsally relative to the lunate
- Again operative reduction is required so analgese, and refer.

⊙ Hand injuries

Fractures

Metacarpal fractures

- Most commonly fractured is the neck of the 5th metacarpal as a result of a punch injury or 'boxer's fracture'
- Deformity, extensor lag, or rotational deformity may be present, although rotational deformity is much more common in proximal or middle phalangeal fractures
- Occasionally, there may be carpo-metacarpal subluxation, which may be subtle both clinically and radiologically. (These can cause significant morbidity and should be referred for specialist opinion)
- Any wound overlying any knuckle should prompt specific questions regarding the aetiology
- A fight bite should be considered as the cause. This will require a thorough examination to ensure no foreign body contaminants, such as fractured teeth
- Irrigation and cleaning of these wounds should take place and referral for X-ray as determined by clinical exam
- Consideration for hepatitis B and C and human immunodeficiency virus (HIV) should be made
- Prophylactic antibiotics should be commenced if a human bite is the cause of the wound, although this is no substitute for thorough cleaning of the wound
- Treatment of uncomplicated wounds rarely requires operative correction and can be managed with a variety of treatments form simple neighbour strapping to a volar slab for 10 days.

Proximal and middle phalangeal fractures

- A common injury in ball games
- Patterns of injury can often be predicted by the mechanism of injury
- Most isolated transverse fractures are stable, but fractures that are oblique or intra-articular are more likely to be unstable
- Clinical examination should help to elicit concerning features such as rotational deformity, which will require correction
- Pitchside treatment involves analgesia and neighbour strapping with referral for X-ray.

Distal phalangeal fractures

- Usually, the result of crush injuries to the tip of the finger such as another player standing on the patient's finger
- Very painful injuries that require splinting to assist pain
- If compound then ensure thorough cleaning and remove the nail if necessary
- Antibiotics prophylactically have been historically given, but are of no proven benefit.

Volar plate injuries
- Occur secondary to hyperextension to the proximal interphalangeal joint
- Common in basketball players and goalkeepers
- Examination reveals a fusiform swelling around the proximal interphalangeal joint (PIPJ) with maximal tenderness over the volar aspect of the joint
- There may be an associated fracture involving the base of the middle phalanx
- These injuries require splinting and reassessment of function after about 10–14 days.

Dislocations

Proximal and distal interphalangeal joint dislocation
- These tend to dislocate with the distal bone dislocated dorsally
- Whilst sportsmen occasionally self-reduce these injuries, there is a risk that the cause of the deformity is due to a displaced fracture rather than dislocation and as such an X-ray is usually advised prior to any reduction
- Volar dislocations are much rarer and are often irreducible and unstable
- Once reduced the PIPJ should be kept in full extension, but the distal interphalangeal joint (DIPJ) left free to minimize the risk of boutonniere deformity.

Flexor tendon rupture
- There are two flexor tendons in each finger
  - Flexor digitorum superficialis (FDS), which flexes the proximal interphalangeal joint
  - Flexor digitorum profundus (FDP), which flexes the distal interphalngeal joint
- Any loss of flexion at either necessitates X-ray and in the case of a wound, surgical exploration
- Due consideration should also be given to exploration to any wound found on the volar aspect of either the palm or fingers even in the absence of loss of function as injury to these areas may result in occult injuries with delayed rupture if not treated.

Mallet injuries
- Common injury—exterior tendon rupture to digital phalanx
- May be innocuous, such as when tying shoelaces or after direct trauma causing forced flexion on an extended finger
- Injuries can be associated with no bony injury on X-ray or associated intra-articular fracture of the base of the distal phalanx
- They require splinting in a mallet splint for a minimum of 6 weeks.

ⓘ Thumb injuries

Bennett's fracture dislocation
- Mechanism of injury is usually forced abduction or direct force along the long axis of the thumb
- It is common in skiers, ballgames, and cyclists
- Results in an intra-articular fracture to the base of the thumb carpometacarpal joint, which is inherently unstable and will require operative fixation.

Ulnar collateral ligament rupture
- Caused by forced abduction of the thumb
- Common is skiers, especially on dry slopes
- Untreated this injury will cause permanent disability by causing interference of grasp
- There will be tenderness and swelling over the ulnar aspect of the metacarpophalangeal joint of the thumb
- Complete rupture paradoxically may not be particularly painful and present with obvious laxity on stressing the joint
- All injuries should be referred for X-ray and definitive treatment—ranging from cast or splint through to operative correction.

Lower limb injury

Lower limb injury

- It is calculated that approximately 40–60% of sport injuries seen in EDs in the UK affect the lower limb.

! The thigh

Femoral fractures

- Large forces are required to break an adult femoral shaft and these injuries are often associated with violent or multisystem trauma
- It is extremely important to exclude other serious injuries, including those to pelvis, hip, and knee
- Pre-existing conditions increasing risks of fracture also need to be considered (e.g. osteoporosis/athletic female triad, metastatic, or other metabolic disease)
- There is usually a shortened externally rotated/abducted hip, severe pain and inability to weight bear. In distal (supracondylar) fractures the gastrocnemius will pull the more distal fragment away from the proximal end.

▶▶ Fractures of the femoral shaft can cause a very fast and life-threatening haemorrhage. This is more pronounced in compound injuries.
- Apply principles of airway, breathing, circulation (ABC) assessment
- Obtain IV access immediately with two large bore cannulae
- Blood should be cross-matched as soon as possible
- Start fluid resuscitation, as this could be a life-threatening haemorrhage
- Give opioid analgesia
- Splinting with Thomas or other traction splints will reduce complications of haemorrhage/fat embolus and will help pain control.

Femoral stress fractures

- Femoral stress fractures are not common, but should be suspected in an athlete who has undergone a sudden increase in their training schedule. The athlete may complain of poorly localized pain in the anterior thigh, which may refer proximally or distally into the knee
- MRI or bone scan may be more sensitive than radiographs in detecting this fracture
- Treatment involves relative offload with conservative management preferred for compression-side fractures and surgical fixation for some tension-side fractures
- Depending on the nature of the fracture, correction of predisposing factors may need to be considered
  - Smoking
  - Athletic female triad
  - Hormonal disturbances and lower limb mechanics have all been associated with stress fractures in the lower limb.

Hamstring origin avulsion

- This is a relatively common injury in adolescents and should be suspected in any athlete in this age group presenting with a hamstring strain. The larger avulsions of the ischial apophysis may be identified by X-ray
- MRI will demonstrate injured bony contours and muscle status with no radiation exposure
- Only displacements of greater than 3 cm are thought to require surgical fixation

- However, if avulsion is detected early referral to orthopaedic specialist is required. Surgical reattachment is becoming increasingly popular and is associated with better outcomes in recent literature
- Avulsion of ischial origin is also seen in adult power lifters and is the result of an award sudden forced hip flexion on an extended knee
- Early surgical intervention has a good prognosis.

Muscle injuries

Although not life-threatening muscle injuries are common and cause considerable time away from sport. They can be classified into grades I–III:
- Grade I is a minor strain with pain on active resisted contraction of the muscle, where the athlete may complete his participation before reporting the injury
- Grade II pain on active unopposed contraction and stretch
- Grade III which is a full thickness tear.

This will be important to the sportsman because it will determine his time to return to sport from anything up to 2 weeks.
- Grade I: 2 weeks
- Grade II: 2–8 weeks.
- Grade III: 8+ weeks for full thickness tears. The rectus femoris (kicking, jumping, sprinting) and hamstring muscles (sprinting, football) are commonly injured.

Emergency treatment of an injured muscle should include ice and compression as soon as possible.
- This minimizes bleeding into the muscle and is thought to reduce scar formation and therefore return to sport or active work time, as well as making a recurrence less likely.
- Referral to a physiotherapist will ensure active graduated return to activity using a progressive functional rehabilitation programme optimizing muscle health and healing.
- Imaging with MRI and ultrasound may be appropriate in the higher-level sportsman.

Quadriceps contusion
- The quadriceps contusion ('dead leg') follows direct impact into the anterior thigh usually by a knee, shoulder, or foot
- The athlete is usually able to continue activity until bleeding increases pressure within the thigh and a dull ache inhibits the affected quadriceps
- There is a diffuse tenderness to palpation over the affected area and range of movement is affected. Vastus intermedius is crushed against the femur and is more commonly affected
- Immediate treatment should be ice and compression to minimize bleeding and time out from sport. This can be days to weeks depending on the force of impact and immediate management of the lesion
- Gentle mobility and range of movement exercises should be encouraged. No imaging is usually required unless a significant muscle tear is suspected.

ⓘ **Knee injuries**

Fractures

Tibial plateau fractures
- Tibial plateau fractures may be seen in high velocity injuries, such as skiing or in low-energy knee twisting mechanisms
- The patient will complain of difficulty in weight bearing and pain
- These fractures need to be excluded in all higher grade collateral ligament injuries
- Radiographs may show obvious fracture or it may be harder to detect if the fracture is undisplaced
- If mechanisms alert the clinician to possibility of fracture a horizontal lateral radiograph may show presence of fat–fluid level (lipohaemathrosis)
- Magnetic resonance imaging (MRI) will show any associated menisceal or anterior cruciate ligament (ACL) injury
- Emergency management involves analgesing and splinting the knee in extension and non-weight bearing crutches
- Conservative treatment is occasionally possible in minimally displaced fractures but arthroscopy may allow direct visualization of articular surfaces and menisci and undetected detached osteochondral fragmentation.

Patellar fractures
- A fracture of the patella usually follows a direct impact onto this sesamoid bone from a fall or from direct contact
- Occasionally, it follows forced and sudden contraction of the quadriceps muscle
- A congenital bipartite patellar can be confused with a fracture and can occur in the lateral upper pole, lateral margin, or inferior pole and can mimic a fracture symptomatically as the impact can disrupt and inflame the synchondrosis
- Anteroposterior (AP) and lateral X-rays will be required and give idea of degree of displacement of fragments
- X-ray of the contralateral side may help exclude bipartite patella as these are rarely unilateral
- Emergency management involves analgesia and splinting the knee
- Patellar fractures should be referred for surgical opinion
- Fractures with minimal displacement, well preserved articular surfaces and intact extensor mechanism can be managed conservatively
- Patellar fractures with overlying skin wounds can undergo delayed fixation and should be covered with antibiotic prophylaxis.

Dislocations

Knee
- The knee joint is a very stable joint and as such dislocations are rare
- When they occur they are usually the results of significant forces such as the tibia being forced backwards in a road traffic accident (RTA) or a fall from height

- Associated injuries should always be sought and the ABC approach followed
- The knee will appear clinically deformed, the athlete in extreme pain
- Neurovascular examination should be carried out to ascertain the associated injuries to both the popliteal artery and the peroneal nerve
- If a vascular deficit is found pitchside then consideration must be given to reducing the dislocation pre hospital. This is usually performed by carrying out longitudinal traction
- This decision will be multifactorial, i.e. having an appropriate medical facility minutes away it may be more appropriate to split the limb as best possible, analgese and immediately transfer
- Imaging both plain film and computed tomography (CT) will be required, and serial vascular assessments should be performed with the patient being required to be admitted for these serial observations
- It should be remembered that significant vascular injury can occur with normal examination of pulses and so vascular assessment will involve some form of investigation whether that be angiography, ankle brachial index, or ultrasonography
- Associated fractures and ligament disruption is almost invariable and surgical management will be dictated by the presence of these findings.

Patellar dislocations/subluxations

- Patellar dislocations most commonly occur laterally and can be atraumatic or traumatic
- Traumatic dislocations will follow a history of significant traumatic force following jumps or rotational movements and are accompanied by haemathrosis and severe pain
- The patients describe popping or 'knee dislocation' and until closer inspection may mimic ACL rupture. The patella may spontaneously reduce, or require analgesia and manipulation
- Examination reveals significant effusion, a tender medial border, tenderness, and apprehension on gentle lateral pressure on the patella
- Athlete may be unable to raise straight leg as active contraction of the quadriceps will be very painful. (Exclude patella tendon rupture or quads tendon rupture by palpation of defects proximal and distal to patella)
- To reduce a patellar dislocation analgese the athlete (Entonox® is ideal) extend the knee, whilst applying gentle pressure to the patella in a medial direction
- Risk factors include generalized ligamentous laxity (hypermobility), genu valgum, patella alta (where the patella sits much more superiorly than normal) and compromise to static stability of the knee. (e.g. dysplastic patella or hypoplastic lateral condyle)
- X-rays should include skyline as well as antero-posterior (AP) lateral and intercondylar views to look for associated osteochondral injuries/ medial patellar facet injuries and resultant loose bodies. MRI will show bone bruising on the lateral femoral condyle and medial patella and it may show a degree of insult to the chondral surfaces or demonstrate loose fragment not detected by radiographs

- First episodes of traumatic patellar dislocations may be treated conservatively. A period of immobilization is a necessity to allow healing of the medial stabilizing structures
- Arthroscopy is indicated in recurrent dislocators (approx 50% of first time dislocators)
- It is also indicated in first patella dislocation for detection/excision or reattachment of osteochondral fragments and detailed inspection of chondral surfaces where a high degree of injury is suspected on MRI
- Additionally allows repair of medial patello-femoral ligament to aid stability.

Tendon ruptures

Patellar tendon ruptures

- Sudden unexpected eccentric contraction of powerful quadriceps muscle, e.g. landing awkwardly, can cause patellar tendon to rupture
- Athletes are usually under the age of 40 and the rupture is more commonly closer to the inferior patella pole
- The athlete will experience localized pain and inability to maintain leg extension and the patellar will be visibly retracted proximally if rupture is complete
- Straight leg raise may be inhibited with pain and effusion in a partial tear.
- Radiographs will demonstrate any bony avulsion and a high riding patella. Ultrasound (US) will show degree of tear if not clinically obvious
- Partial tears may be treated conservatively with 3–6 weeks immobilization, but experienced surgical opinion may be warranted to determine whether remaining tendon will cope with functional load in an athletic population
- Tears need early surgical reconstruction as repair less successful if late.

Quadriceps tendon ruptures

- Quadriceps tendon ruptures will usually happen in the older athletes or those with associated systemic conditions such as gout, diabetes, hyperthyroidism, or renal failure
- It is more common in males and may be partial or full thickness
- The athlete is unable to walk or extend his leg
- Knee flexion may be intact if pain permits
- Quadriceps rupture is usually extremely painful
- A haemathrosis will develop and a defect may be palpable usually just proximal to the patellar
- The defect may not be immediately obvious with a tense haemathrosis Surgical correction is required within 48 h to obtain a good result
- Radiographs will show a low lying patella and MRI will demonstrate extent of tear.

Meniscal injuries

- Usually, the result of a twisting knee injury with a foot anchored on the ground. Classically, the effusion develops over 24 h, although no effusion may develop
- The athlete may feel a significant amount of pain and hear a snap, tear, or may feel nothing

- This injury is usually associated with joint line tenderness
- A positive McMurray test with reproduction of pain or 'a clunk' on combined flexion and rotation of the tibia makes meniscal injury more likely
- The older athlete may have a greater predisposition following degenerative change with a relatively small trauma
- More severe meniscal injuries with pain and restriction of range/fixed flexion may occur in bucket handle tears as displaced meniscal fragments may prevent normal articular movement. This should prompt rapid arthroscopy
- Look for chondral involvement +/– ACL involvement in the more traumatic injuries.

Ligament injuries

Anterior cruciate ligament injuries

- ACL injury can happen as a result of a sudden deceleration, rotation, jump, or by any fall on the athletes flexed knee
- Typically occurs in football, basketball, or skiing, but can happen in any sport reproducing the injury mechanism described
- More commonly there will be a tense haemathrosis developing over a couple of hours, but there may be little swelling especially if previous insult to the ligament may have rendered few fibres intact by the time of the complete disruption
- The athlete will normally be unable to continue participation in the activity due to the pain:
  - They may describe a snapping or crack and occasionally describe the knee 'going out of its normal position'
  - You may have a window to examine effectively if pain permits immediately after injury
  - Examination is more difficult and less accurate for several days once haemathrosis, pain, and muscle spasm take hold
- Lachmans test is both more sensitive and specific than anterior drawer test:
  - Remember to compare to contralateral side, as different degrees of laxity may be normal to any individual athlete
  - Pivot shift is very effective in demonstrating torn ACL in a very relaxed athlete
- ACL can be accompanied by meniscal injuries, collateral ligament rupture, or a Segond fracture where there is an avulsion just distal to the lateral tibial plateau
- The pivot shift may be absent in the presence of tear of the medial collateral ligament and beware of capsular tears where effusions may leak out of the torn capsule confusing the clinician away from serious internal derangement of the knee
- Good history taking is important.

Lachmans test

- Lie the athlete supine
- Flex the injured knee to 20–30°

- Place one hand behind the tibia with the thumb coming round the front of the lower leg to rest on the tibial tuberosity
- Place the other hand above the knee and attempt to pull the lower leg anteriorly
- A definite end point should be felt and this should be compared with the unaffected knee.

Posterior cruciate ligament (PCL) injuries

- This classically occurs as an RTA injury where the tibia is translated posteriorly under force
- In sport it will usually happen in a hyperextension injury
- Unless posterolateral corner structures are involved the degree of posterior translation is usually minimal and therefore most noticeable at 90° flexion (compare with contralateral side) with a relaxed quadriceps muscle
- Examination would reveal tibial posterior sag/reverse Lachmans and posterior drawer
- Thorough examination of the posterolateral corner is important
- X-rays can aid bony avulsion or other associated fractures that may need urgent surgical intervention
- MRI will help confirm diagnosis
- Isolated posterior collateral ligament (PCL) injuries tend to do well conservatively, but follow-up needs to be done to exclude associated posterolateral corner injuries when patient is pain free
- Rehabilitation will be essential in order to compensate for the posterior instability.

Medial collateral ligament injuries.

Usually sustained after a valgus strain to the knee. They can be classified in terms of severity into three grades:
- Grade 1 (tenderness, pain on valgus stress but no laxity at 30° flexion)
- Grade 2 (tenderness over the ligament, pain, and laxity at 30° flexion but a solid end feel, usually accompanied by swelling)
- Grade 3 (laxity at 30° flexion with no end feel. There may be a sensation of instability, but less pain following the injury since all fibres are in theory disrupted)
- The higher the severity the longer the healing time (approx 2 weeks for grade 1 to >8 weeks for grade 3)
- MRI will confirm diagnosis and will aid the clinician in excluding associated cruciate ligament injuries if clinically difficult due to pain
- Most of these injuries will do well conservatively if given time and the resulting laxity is controlled by the use of a splint. Surgical intervention is required for persistent laxity beyond the prescribed healing period.

Lateral collateral ligament injuries

These injuries are less common than medial collateral ligament (MCL) injuries. Posterolateral corner injuries/instability should be considered for all lateral collateral ligament injuries, as these will require surgical intervention.

ⓘ Leg injuries

Fractures

Tibia and fibular fractures

Rotational injuries in most lower limb dominant sports can result in comminuted (usually spiral) fractures of the tibia and fibula. Direct trauma may also result in fractures.

- The athlete will be in pain
- Swelling and deformity are usually obvious
- Do not be distracted by the lower limb injury, and exclude other life-threatening injuries first using the ABC approach
- Open fractures need immediate cover with sterile, moist swabs soaked in saline/water and splintage. A photograph of the wound is useful to stop repeated removal of the dressing.
- Check tetanus cover and arrange immediate hospital referral.
- Immobilization will help pain, and opioid analgesia may be required.

The popliteal artery can be injured following proximal tibial fractures, and the common peroneal nerve can complicate a proximal fibula fracture so lateral foot sensation and foot dorsiflexion should be documented during assessment. All tibial and fibula fractures can further be complicated by emergent compartment syndromes so careful neurovascular observation should follow in the hours and days following these fractures. The deep peroneal nerve can be assessed by testing sensation between the first and second toes.

Maisonneuve fracture

- This is an ascending fracture of the shaft or proximal fibula
- It follows a severe ankle ligament injury where the ankle syndesmosis is disrupted and therefore unstable
- There may be an associated medial malleolus fracture
- Fibular examination should follow all severe ankle injuries
- Syndesmosis injuries are discussed under ankle injuries.

Stress fracture of the tibia

- Tibial stress fracture can present with gradual or sudden shin pain and are located on the tibial medial border.
- Posterior cortex fractures can present with calf pain and history can be confused with a gastro-soleus muscle injury.
- A palpable lump may be felt around the area of the fracture if anterior and chronic.
- Radiographs may miss subtle stress fractures unless they are more chronic in nature. MRI or bone scan and CT will be more sensitive.
- Biomechanics (rigid pes cavus, over-pronated foot), sudden increase in training schedule or change of surface, athletic female triad, hormonal or metabolic disorders should be screened for and addressed.
- Longitudinal stress fractures occur in the distal third of the tibia and have a better prognosis. Stress fractures of the anterior cortex have

a poorer prognosis and can be career ending due to non-union and progression to fracture.
- The athlete should be removed from aggravating activity and risks explained since symptoms will quickly settle.
- The athlete can be offloaded with crutches and an orthotic boot.
- Referral to a specialist with experience in dealing with stress fractures in athletes should be sought early.

Fibular stress fractures
- Usually associated with abnormal foot biomechanics increasing the tractional load of the peroneal muscles.
- Athlete is locally tender at the site of injury but will usually be able to weight bear.
- Relative offload in orthotic boot and referral for biomechanics assessment will usually allow adequate healing.

Muscle injury

Gastrocnemius/soleus
- The gastrocnemius muscle can be injured when landing forward or during a sudden start to a run or jump
- The medial belly is most commonly injured
- Plantar flexion may be painful and the athlete may require crutches
- A heel raise may help alleviate symptoms and allow earlier weight bearing.

Soleus injuries may happen insidiously during a run or landing after a jump.
- They can be differentiated from a gastrocnemius injury when stretching of the calf with the knee in flexion reproduces pain.
- Emergency treatment of calf muscles should involve early ice and compression as previously described for the muscles of the thigh.

① Ankle injuries

Ankle fractures

Lateral malleolus
- Very common injury in sport resulting usually from an inversion injury
- Depending on the type of fracture, the athlete may be able to carry on playing and only complain of pain after ceasing activity
- Examination should be based on the Ottawa ankle guidelines, which have a high sensitivity in excluding bony injury (see 📖 p.249)
- Examination will identify bony tenderness over the lateral malleolus. The medial malleolus should also be palpated as should the entire lower leg paying particular attention to the head and neck of fibula
- Bruising and swelling may be apparent immediately, but may take time to develop
- X-ray will usually reveal the fracture with treatment depending on a number of factors including association of medial malleolar or posterior malleolar fractures
- The fracture can be classified using the Weber classification where:
  - Type A—usually stable injuries with the fracture below the mortice line
  - Type B—spiral fracture starting at the level of the mortice. Potentially unstable depending on associated medial ligamentous or bony injury
  - Type C—fracture above the level of the mortice with associated instability
- Stable fractures may require very little treatment other than symptomatic support whether in a cast or rigid boot. Unstable fractures may require open reduction and internal fixation.

Medial malleolus
- Less common than lateral fractures
- May occur in isolation, but are more commonly associated with lateral malleolar fractures
- Again, examination using the Ottawa guidelines will detect these fractures
- If a medial malleolar fracture is suspected, examination should proceed to look for an associated injury that would render the ankle complex unstable, such as a proximal fibula fracture or injury to the syndesmosis
- Immediate management is as for lateral malleolar fracture, including ice, analgesia as required, and immobilization prior to X-ray.

Talar dome osteochondral injuries
- Ankle ligament injuries can often be associated with talar dome lesions
- Unless considerable in size and, therefore, higher in grade these may be undetected in plain X-ray
- The mechanism usually involves compression to the medial or lateral talus by the tibial plafond
- Talar dome osteochondral injuries can be graded on a scale of I–IV depending on severity

- MRI and CT scanning will allow grading of an osteochondral injury of the ankle. Grade I–II can usually be treated conservatively with a period of offload
- Arthroscopy is warranted for higher grades, which may warrant microfracture and/or removal of loose bodies depending on the degree of severity.

Lateral and posterior talar process fractures

- Posterior talar process fractures can occur in forced plantar flexion and may require 6-week cast immobilization or excision
- Lateral talar process fractures occur in forced dorsiflexion and inversion producing shearing forces into the talus by the calcaneus
- Often confused with lateral ligament sprain. Athlete will present with pain and tenderness anterior and inferior to tip of lateral malleolus, and difficulty with persistent weight-bearing
- The athletes may experience difficulty with prolonged weight-bearing, particularly if fracture extends into posterior facet of subtalar joint
- Mortise view will demonstrate the fracture especially in 20–25° of plantar flexion
- Radiographs can underestimate fragment size
- Further investigation by CT is recommended for accurate sizing and extension of fracture
- Fractures with more than 2 mm displacement or larger than 1 cm are treated surgically as risk of non-union is high
- Conservative treatment involves immobilization in non-weight bearing cast for 4–6 weeks.

Talar stress fractures

- Stress fractures of the talus usually involve the posterolateral aspect
- They are most commonly seen in track, field athletes, and footballers
- Swelling and pain may vary from inability to weight bear to asymptomatic MRI appearances
- CT is required to establish extent of fracture
- Treatment involves cast immobilization and correction of predisposing factors, e.g. over-pronation, athletic triad.

Ankle dislocation

⚠ A potentially catastrophic injury for an athlete, and should be considered as an orthopaedic emergency.

- Usually associated with a fracture of the ankle, but not always
- The ankle can dislocate in a number of different directions, but posteriorly is the most common with the talus forced backwards in relation to the tibia
- Immediate management as always should exclude more significant injuries via the ABC approach
- The athlete will require analgesia—Entonox® is ideal until IV access is gained to allow administration of opioids if available
- Assessment should focus on diagnosis and identification of an associated neurovascular compromise and/or possible compromise to the overlying skin from displaced bone causing tethering

- If these issues are found, then pitchside reduction will be required unless there is a very short transport time to the nearest ED
- Reduction involves manual traction to the ankle usually best achieved by holding the heel in one hand with the other hand on the dorsum of the foot and pulling in a distal direction. Counter traction should be applied proximally, ideally with the athlete's knee flexed to reduce hamstring resistance
- Once reduced splint and transfer
- Cover any compound injury with saline soaks and splint. A photograph avoids repeated removal of the dressing
- Further management will be directed on the associated injuries found post-reduction.

▶ X-ray should confirm the reduction and are not required to be taken prior to the reduction taking place in the ED.

Tendon injuries

Achilles tendon rupture
- Complete or incomplete ruptures are more likely in athletes after the age of 30
- It may occur in a tendon with previous painful tendinopathy or may occur in a tendon previously asymptomatic
- The acute rupture is not always painful
- There may be an audible snap as the tendon tears and athlete may describe 'being struck on the back of the leg'
- There is usually a reduction in function
- On examination the acute swelling may vary.
- Squeezing of the calf may still plantar flex the foot (Simmonds's test) in a partial rupture but the degree of plantar flexion may be diminished on comparison to the contralateral side
- Complete tears will usually leave a palpable defect unless haematoma fills in the gap
- MRI and US will aid the clinician in establishing the degree of tear, but surgical exploration may be warranted even in partially torn tendons to establish the percentage of torn segment
- Longitudinal tears of the tendon may be more easily missed on imaging
- A surgical opinion is warranted early in an athlete. It is generally accepted that surgical repair is advisable for active individuals performing at a higher functional level.

Tibialis posterior ruptures
- An athlete with tibialis posterior rupture will present with a flattened foot arch (compare to contralateral foot) and pain in the navicular tubercle, often extending posteriorly and proximally behind the tibia
- Absence or defect in the tendon may be palpated and will be detected by US and MRI
- Surgical reconstruction is required to restore normal foot arch and power/control in lower limb dominant sports.

Tibialis posterior dislocation

- Dislocation of the tibialis posterior tendon can occur in a forceful dorsiflexion and inversion of the foot
- There is some pain and swelling in the area as the aponeurosis is torn
- The subluxed tendon can be palpated anterior to the medial malleolus
- MRI will demonstrate oedema around the injured area and dynamic ultrasound can demonstrate the subluxing tendon
- Early surgical reconstruction is required in the elite athlete (typically a ballet dancer).

Ligament injuries

Lateral ligament injuries

- Usually caused by a forced inversion lateral ligament. Injuries are very common in a numerous number of sports
- Mechanism can involve a degree of plantar flexion and, therefore, the anterior talo-fibular ligament is usually torn before the calcaneofibular ligament
- Clinical picture depends on severity of the injury and the athlete may be able to finish their event or need assistance in leaving the field
- Swelling may develop immediately or over several hours and compression and ice will reduce degree of swelling and may therefore assist rehabilitation
- Ottawa ankle rules offer the physician a guide as to when to image is required and have a sensitivity of approximately 98%
- Once fracture is excluded, grading can give a guide to prognosis and return to sport:
  - *Grade I:* no ligament laxity
  - *Grade II:* some laxity (compare to contralateral side) but solid endpoint
  - *Grade III:* laxity without endpoint
- More severe grades may benefit from MRI/follow-up to exclude missed osteochondral lesions or fractures.

Deltoid injuries

- The deltoid ligament is better thought of as a complex of ligaments stronger than lateral ligaments in combination. It is probably more commonly injured than previously thought
- The more commonly described injury follows a forced high-energy eversion of the ankle and the athlete is usually unable to weight bear
- There will be immediate emerging swelling and the ankle may be dislocated
- Radiographs can show associated fractures of fibular syndesmosis and talar dome. Occasionally associated with lateral ligament injuries
- MRI and US may show oedema and ligament disruption
- Disruption of the anterior deltoid part of the complex in dancers and footballers following a combined dorsiflexion external rotation insult may cause instability in the anteromedial ankle causing ongoing pain when injury mechanism is reproduced
- They will be varying degrees of tenderness and swelling over the anterior deltoid area
- Surgical exploration may be warranted with continuing pain around the medial ankle as imaging may be deceiving and surgical correction may be required.

Syndesmosis injuries

- Tears of the anterior inferior tibio-fibular ligament can occur within sports involving repeated rotation of the ankle joint (e.g. football, rugby). History of 'tackle from behind' or direct impact to the distal fibula will often precede this injury
- The athlete will generally be unable to continue participation
- There will be some difficulty weight bearing although they can usually progress to walking once the initial pain subsides
- Minor sprains will generally be able to continue playing
- The athlete will describe high ankle pain. High ankle swelling will develop after several hours but may not be marked or may travel distally confusing the clinician onto thinking there is lateral ankle ligament injury
- Pain will be reproduced by combination of ankle dorsiflexion and external rotation
- Palpation of the ligament will usually be painful. Mortise and lateral view will be normal
- Stress diastases views will reveal a separation of the tibia and fibula
- MRI is good at detecting the extent of syndesmosis injury and instability
- Instability should be surgically repaired because of the danger of future arthritis
- Additionally, athletes requiring high rotational stability will be unable to progress to normal functional levels
- Traditional methods of syndesmosis repair by screw fixation are slowly being replaced by tightrope repair
- This is favoured in an athletic population due to earlier return to sport secondary to decreased ankle stiffness during rehabilitation and less morbidity associated with metalwork in the area
- Syndesmosis injuries can be associated with medial malleolar fractures.

⚠ Foot injuries

Fractures

Base of fifth metatarsal fractures

Two types of fractures are commonly described at the base of fifth metatarsal.

- The peroneus brevis tendon attaches to the base of the fifth metatarsal and may avulse a fragment in inversion injuries:
  - This fracture may be associated with a lateral ankle ligament injury
  - There can be involvement of the metatarso-cuboid articular surface
  - This fracture has a good prognosis when treated conservatively by offload and immobilization (3–6 weeks) followed by graduated return to loading
  - This fracture is not to be confused with the normal apophysis of the 9–14 age-group (Apophyseal line runs parallel to metatarsal shaft)
- A fracture seen more distally, 1.5 cm distal to the metatarsal tubercle, at the diaphyses (Jones fracture) disrupts blood supply to the displaced fragment
- This is associated with a poorer prognosis and will often require internal fixation especially in the athletic population where quick return to sport can be associated with non-union.

Calcaneal fractures

- These usually occur after a fall from height. The majority are intra-articular as a result of axial loading, whilst 30% are extra-articular and can be associated with rotational forces being applied to the hindfoot
- Axial load type fractures are associated with spinal fractures in up to 15% so these injuries need to be excluded and should be assumed until proven otherwise
- Clinical examination will reveal tenderness on squeezing the heel, with likely swelling and bruising (though these may be delayed signs)
- Immediate management will involve splinting the ankle with analgesia appropriate to manage the patient's symptoms
- Compartment syndrome due to swelling should be regularly assessed for, and the foot elevated and iced
- Orthopaedic management will be directed by the findings on plain film, with reconstructed CT images playing a more frequent role in determining treatment.

Anterior calcaneal process fracture

- The anterior calcaneal process can be injured in avulsion (more commonly) and compression
- Avulsion fractures occur after combined adduction and plantar flexion that results in avulsion of the anterior process by the bifurcate ligament
- Compression fractures follow forced forefoot abduction where calcaneus and cuboid are compressed against each other
- There is resulting tenderness just anterior to the sinus tarsi opening, anterior and inferior to the anterior tibio-fibular ligament, distinguishing this injury from lateral ankle ligament sprains

- Lateral hindfoot and, lateral oblique views of the ankle will best demonstrate this fracture but MRI may be necessary
- These fractures require immobilization in below knee cast for 4 weeks if picked up early and conservative treatment is possible depending on the size of the fragment. Refer for orthopaedic opinion.

Calcaneal stress fractures

- More commonly seen in those walking unaccustomed to the load or marching this is usually an insidious onset injury. The athlete complains of heel pain and is tender on calcaneal squeeze test
- Radiographs may show sclerotic appearances if the injury has been present for some time. Prognosis is generally good following a period of relative offload.

Navicular stress fractures

- Navicular stress fractures can present with midfoot pain and swelling
- The athlete may report 'aching' present for some time, but worse after a particular activity
- Since this condition can be associated with a poor outcome for the future career of the athlete, tenderness over the navicular should be treated and investigated as a stress fracture until this condition is excluded
- Radiographs are not sensitive, so CT and MRI are recommended for diagnosis and evaluation
- Non-weight-bearing immobilization is required, after which tenderness is re-assessed
- This provides the clinician with a good opportunity to attempt to correct risk factors, which include reduced range of motion in the ankle, athletic female triad, and over-pronation
- CT may additionally provide more accurate evaluation of a co-existing tarsal coalition.

Lisfranc fracture dislocation

The tarsometatarsal joint (Lisfranc joint) may be dislocated dorsally when a high-energy impact is sustained on a plantar flexed foot through an axial plane. Even without associated fractures this injury is career-ending if untreated due to complications of mid-foot collapse and post-traumatic arthritis.

- Compartment syndrome of the foot is also associated with this condition
- There will be a history of significant traumatic episode and the athlete will complain of midfoot pain, and may or may not be able to weight bear
- Swelling will develop over the midfoot and the Lisfranc joint will be tender to palpation
- Pain can be reproduced by abduction and pronation of the forefoot over a fixed hindfoot
- Blood supply may be compromised in severe injuries as dorsalis pedis may be injured or compressed
- The Lisfranc injury may not be immediately obvious on X-rays, as spontaneous reduction of the joint may have taken place. Fractures at

the base of second metatarsal and anterior cuboid may be evident, and should suggest a Lisfranc dislocation
- Weight-bearing views may help in demonstrating relationship between first and second metatarsal, but may not be well tolerated by the individual
- MRI and CT may be required
- If no gross instability remains in a less severe injury 6 weeks of below knee immobilization is required
- Observation of neurovascular supply should be maintained for several weeks
- Precise anatomical reduction required and this often involves open reduction internal fixation (ORIF)
- Note that dislocations without a fracture often have a poorer outcome despite ORIF.

Sesamoid injuries

Fractures
- Located within the flexor hallucis brevis the sesamoid bones confer mechanical advantage to this tendon, and assist weight bearing across the 1st metatarso-phalangeal (MTP)
- Fractures usually involve the medial sesamoid
- The onset may be sudden or more insidious in nature and may follow forefoot weight bearing activities or sudden landing
- Swelling is limited but direct palpation over the affected bone is excruciatingly tender
- AP lateral and oblique, as well as axial sesamoid views will identify the fracture
- Bipartatite medial sesamoids could be confused with fracture where edges are usually irregular in the latter
- MRI can be helpful
- Treatment includes immobilization in non-weight-bearing cast
- Loading should be returned gradually and the sesamoid should be offloaded with orthotics, as this is a fatigue fracture
- Excision of the sesamoid is used when conservative approaches fail, but is not recommended in the athlete. It is associated with development of hallux valgus (if medial sesamoid resected) or halux varus (if lateral resected)
- Excision has also been associated with cock-up/claw toe deformity and first MTP stiffness.

Sesamoiditis
- Trauma, infection vascular, necrosis, and systemic inflammatory conditions can all cause inflammation of the sesamoids
- Sesamoid shape may also influence the amount of soft tissue micro-trauma that they cause in surrounding tissues when loading
- Radiograph sesamoid views and MRI will help distinguish from other conditions affecting the sesamoids
- Treatment requires offload and orthotic prescription
- Infiltration with corticosteroid may help accelerate the recovery from symptoms as mechanical causes are corrected
- Excision should be avoided for reasons listed above.

ⓘ **Ottawa Foot and Ankle Guidelines**

These validated guidelines have a sensitivity of about 98% in excluding a fracture to the ankle or foot after injury.

Ankle

X-rays are only required if there is any pain in the ankle region (between the malleoli) and any one of the following:

- Bone tenderness along the distal 6 cm of the posterior edge of the tibia or tip of the medial, malleolus *or*
- Bone tenderness along the distal 6 cm of the posterior edge of the fibula or tip of the lateral malleolus *or*
- An inability to bear weight both immediately and in the ED for four steps.

Foot

X-rays are only required if there is any pain in the area of the midfoot and any one of the following:

- Bone tenderness at the base of the fifth metatarsal (for foot injuries), *or*
- Bone tenderness at the navicular bone (for foot injuries), *or*
- An inability to bear weight both immediately and in the ED for four steps.

Further reading

Stiell IG, Greenberg GH, McKnight RD, et al. (1993). Decision rules for the use of radiography in acute ankle injuries. Refinement and prospective validation. *J Am Med Ass* **269**: 1127–32.

Paediatrics

Introduction

The United Nations Convention on the Rights of a Child states that a child is considered 'every human being below the age of eighteen years'. This definition has been accepted by all 4 UK governments.

We all have a social responsibility to encourage children to participate in sport, whether that be in our roles as doctors, physiotherapists, teachers, or most importantly parents. The benefits of regular exercise in the long-term health of a population should be built on a foundation that promotes that regular exercise should be undertaken at as young an age as possible.

Children should not, however, be viewed simply as small adults. There are many differences that should be considered in ensuring that children are enabled to exercise in a safe environment.

- Physical (anatomical)
- Physiological
- Pathological
- Psychological
- Protection.

We shall look at these different areas to highlight the kind of problems that may be encountered.

⚠ Note in the presentation of cardiac arrest please refer to 📖 p.82.

⚠ Note in the presentation of anaphylaxis please refer to 📖 p.96.

Physical (anatomical)

All children develop and grow at different rates and these weights and heights are charted on plots giving centile measurements. These charts demonstrate the great differences in weight and height between children at the same age or in the same class at school. Growth spurts tend to occur around puberty—with girls usually commencing puberty slightly earlier than boys. These changing physical characteristics can play a part in affecting the psychological development of a child, especially if a child develops particularly early or late in comparison with their peers.

Physical differences play an important part in the injury rates of children. Rugby is a sport that recognizes the potential difference in physical size between children at different ages and the problems that can arise as a result of this. As such, there is a graded introduction into this game using smaller pitches and 'touch', rather than tackle-based games.

Analgesia is prescribed usually on a weight basis. Most over the counter medications such as paracetamol or ibuprofen will have a dosage regime on the side of the bottle, but for more precise dosing, it is important to measure or calculate the child's weight to prevent under- or over-dosing. This is highly important in the prescription and administration of any drug and not just analgesia.

In situations of critical illness, such as epilepsy or cardiac arrest where time is especially pressing, knowledge of the child's weight will allow accurate calculation, and aid administration of medications timeously and safely.

Various formulae have been used to calculate a child's weight, based on age. As long as the child is between the ages of 1 and 13 years old the following formula can be used:

$$Weight (kg) = (Age \times 3) + 7$$

For example, a 6-year-old would be estimated to weigh 25 kg.

⚠ Remember this is a rough estimate.

Physiological

Children's physiology changes remarkably as they grow. Respiratory rate, heart rate, blood pressure (BP) will continue to change until adult levels are reached. This is important when trying to assess an injured child and interpret their clinical condition. Realizing that it can be normal for a child to have a resting pulse rate of 120 bpm and a respiratory rate of 20 bpm can have a major impact on how you proceed in your management.

Paediatric brain physiology is similar to that of adults in terms of cerebral autoregulation and perfusion pressures. Children tend to have a lower cerebral perfusion pressure than adults but this is offset by their lower BP.

Different to adults, however, children can become much more easily hypovolaemic and this can occur due to blood loss from scalp wounds—much less common in adults.

⚠ Children usually have a marked physiological reserve and can appear to be coping up until the point where they decompensate dramatically.

See Table 18.1 for a range of normal findings (Wyatt et al., 2006, p. 629).

Table 18.1 Normal (expected) physiological values at different ages*

Age (years)	Respiratory rate	Heart rate	Systolic BP
<1	30–40	110–160	70–90
1–2	25–35	100–150	80–95
2–5	25–30	95–140	80–100
5–12	20–25	80–120	90–110
>12	15–20	60–100	100–120

Expected systolic BP = 80 + (age in years x 2) mmHg.

Adapted from the American Academy of Pediatrics and the American College of Emergency Physicians, 2004, 2007. Used with permission.

Pathological

As a result of the physical differences between the immature and adult skeleton, different types of pathologies and fractures can arise. The following fractures are specific to children for example:

- *Torus (Buckle):* typically stable injuries that can be treated usually by a wrist splint. May be very little to find clinically
- *Greenstick:* a break in one cortex and a bend in the other. May be unstable and change position. Manipulation may be required. Cast minimum treatment
- *Epiphyseal:* the Salter Harris classification describes the 5 different fractures that can affect the growth plates. Management depends on the extent of the injury, but these can cause considerable morbidity
- *Plastic bowing:* an uncommon injury that usually occurs in association with a second fracture that is the cause of the shortening, i.e. distal radius fracturing and resulting bowing of the ulna.

Fractures are just one example of the differences in pathology that will be suffered by a child. There are many others that should be borne in mind, including childhood illnesses, such as chickenpox, which may affect both the child athlete and potentially his classmates too if undetected.

Psychological

- Children need to be allowed to develop both physically and psychologically
- Care needs to be taken to provide an appropriate environment for exercise to take place
- This includes appropriate areas both for training, playing, and changing
- Adequate supervision needs to take place at all times, whilst balancing the issues of privacy.

Bullying can take many forms, but at its most basic, it is either physical or non-physical, where either may be absolutely intolerable and devastating for the child. It may originate from other children, but occasionally from adults as well. Pressure to succeed felt by the touchline parent may be directed towards a child who they see as underperforming. This is clearly unacceptable, and may inhibit the child and hinder them from wanting to participate in any form of exercise in the future.

Children must be treated as individuals. They must be encouraged foremost to participate in exercise and, thereafter, to maximize their potential. This takes a great deal of skill and patience to get the best out of each child. Whatever problems that may prevent or delay a child from participating in sport, such as extreme self-consciousness should be sought for and addressed.

Protection

Child protection is an area that should never be compromised when dealing with children and sport. It is encumbant on any health professional to consider issues relating to child protection when presented with a child seeking medical attention. Any injury sustained by a child should have an adequate explanation to accompany it. Sport can be used as a convenient excuse to explain away an injury and whilst in the overwhelming majority of patients this will be an appropriate explanation, other factors should always be in the back of the clinicians mind.

- Delay in presentation
- Recurrent unexplained injury
- Unusual patterns of injury
- Withdrawn child
- Multiple attendances to Emergency Department (EDs)
- Unusual time of attendance to EDs.

These factors are just some of the many red flags that may present to the team physician. It should be remembered that the difficulty in identifying a child with child protection issues lies in that a child may present with all the red flags and have absolutely no issues, or present with none of the red flags and be at risk. Herein lies the problem. In order to mitigate risk it is vital that any adult dealing with children has undertaken adequate training in child protection issues and had an adequate assessment made of themselves according to local policies and procedures.

Help, advice, and information may be sought from the child's GP, health visitor, school nurse, or social work team.

Statutory guidance is available in England via *Working Together to Safeguard children 2010*, whilst in Scotland the Protection of Children (Scotland) Act 2003 also provides guidance.

⚠ 'If you don't consider it, you will miss it.'—is an adage that holds true in all medical disciplines, but is never more important than in the assessment of child protection.

☠ Choking child

- Children may choke at any age, although it is more common in younger children.
- If the presentation has been witnessed then the diagnosis is usually clearly apparent and the algorithm below can be followed.
- In cases where the event is not witnessed, a high index of suspicion should be given in any child who suddenly develops:
  - Cyanosis
  - Drooling
  - Stridor
  - Clutching throat
  - Dyspnoea
  - Wheeze
  - Intractable coughing
  - Silent chest.

Differential diagnoses of this presentation therefore includes anaphylaxis, asthma, and epiglottitis. The sudden nature of the onset of the airway obstruction, however, is key in making the diagnosis.

Management

The initial management follows the flow diagram in Fig. 18.1.

- Assessment is made as to whether the child has an effective cough or not
- If they are able to cough and shift air into the lungs then leave them in a position of comfort. They should be encouraged to cough and regularly checked to ensure no deterioration
- If the cough is ineffective then check the child's consciousness level. If they are unconscious then open the airway, perform 5 rescue breaths and start cardiopulmonary resuscitation (CPR). If they are conscious then perform 5 back blows followed by 5 abdominal thrusts (or 5 chest thrusts if the child is under 1-year-old)
- Back blows are performed by striking the child between the scapula. After each blow, check to see if the foreign body has become dislodged
- Abdominal thrusts are performed by standing behind the child. Make a fist and place this hand between the child's umbilicus and xiphisternum. Place the other hand on-top of the closed fist, and pull sharply inwards and upwards
- Chest thrusts are performed with the hands in the same position as for CPR, but with a rate in the region of 1 s per thrust.

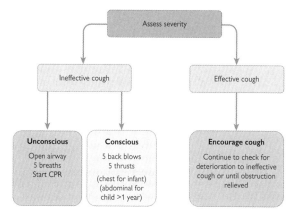

Fig. 18.1 Choking child algorithm. Reproduced with the kind permission of the Resuscitation Council (UK).

:Ö: Asthma

The incidence of asthma is on the increase especially in the paediatric population.

The classic presentation is wheeze, breathlessness, and cough. There may be a history of atopy or nocturnal coughing. Acute asthma attacks are relatively common and usually resolve with inhalation of a short-acting beta-2 agonist. In situations where the child deteriorates, treatment should be carried out as detailed below.

The differential diagnosis differs slightly in children compared with adults where children are more prone to choking, and this should be remembered and considered. Other potential causes of shortness of breath, such as anaphylaxis, pneumothorax, and pneumonia are also potential differentials.

Management of asthma is similar to that of adults in that the exacerbation should be classified into one of the categories below depending on the features found on assessment. The age of the child is also taken into account. The remainder of this chapter refers to the management of a child over 5 years old. (As per Scottish Intercollegiate Guidelines Network (SIGN) guidelines 101).

Initial pre-hospital treatment involves administration of a beta-agonist such as salbutamol. 2 puffs should be given every 2 min (preferably via a spacer).

Criteria for referring to hospital
- More than 10 puffs of salbutamol required
- Any features of acute severe or life-threatening as detailed in Box 18.1.

Treatment of acute asthma
- Sit the child up to aid lung expansion and reassure
- Assess and classify into one of the 3 categories in Box 18.1. Note that peak exploratory flow rate (PEFR) is vital
- Note past medical history; risk of severity increases with past history of hospital admission for asthma, ventilation, >3 types of asthma drugs and repeated presentations to the Emergency Department (ED)
- Initial management is with inhaled bronchodilators (e.g. salbutamol) 2 puffs every 2 min then reassess, including PEFR
- If there are any features of a severe or life-threatening exacerbation, or SaO_2 <94% then commence oxygen at as high a flow rate as possible—ideally 15 L/min via non-rebreathable facemask (CO_2 retention is never an issue at this stage)
- In all cases of acute asthma give po prednisolone 30–40 mg, usually for 3 days
- A nebulizer should be used, if available, in any child with an acute severe or life-threatening exacerbation. If there is a poor response to beta agonist add ipratropium bromide to the nebulized beta agonist

Box 18.1 Acute severe and life-threatening features

Moderate exacerbation
- Increasing symptoms
- PEF between 50 and 75% of best or predicted
- No features of acute severe asthma

Acute severe exacerbation
Any ONE of:
- PEF between 33 and 50%
- SaO_2 <92%
- Cannot complete sentences in one breath or too breathless to feed/talk
- Pulse >125 bpm
- Respiration >30 bpm

Life-threatening exacerbation
Any ONE of:
- PEF <33% or unable to carry out
- SaO_2 <92%
- Silent chest
- Poor respiratory effort
- Cyanosed
- Hypotensive
- Exhausted
- Coma

⚠ Bradycardia is a pre-terminal event.

☠ Seizures

See 📖 p.38 and 98.

Seizures can occur in children for many reasons. Some of these such as febrile convulsions are unique to children and do not occur in adults.

Causes of seizures in children

- Epilepsy
- Trauma—head injury
- Infection
- Hypoglycaemia
- Febrile convulsions
- Cerebral palsy
- Congenital.

This list is not exhaustive. Best management is based on prevention so ensure you are up to date with each athlete's medication if they are known to fit. Focus of management of epilepsy or seizures of any aetiology is clearly prevention. When a seizure occurs, the management is prescriptive. Being prepared is vital—ensure you have access to the correct equipment including a mobile phone.

Status epilepticus is defined as seizure activity, ongoing for more than 30 min, or repeated seizures without consciousness being regained. It is a life-threatening condition with a high mortality, the rate of which increases with the increasing duration of the seizure.

Management aims

- Maintain an airway
- Terminate the seizure if not self-terminated within 2 min
- Identify potential reversible causes namely hypoglycaemia.

⚠ Remember that cardiac arrest caused by ventricular fibrillation may present as a short-lived seizure. Check for a pulse in all patients suffering from a seizure.

When to phone an ambulance

- Status epilepticus
- Seizure lasting longer than 5 min
- Athletes first seizure
- Seizure as a result of injury
- Injury resulting from seizure
- Multiple seizures.

Medications

There are a number of medications belonging to the benzodiazepine family that can be used to terminate seizures.

All members of the benzodiazepine family have a similar side-effect profile, such as respiratory depression and hypotension. The extent of these effects varies between drugs, but being familiar with these effects is paramount, as is having the correct equipment to deal with them when they arise.

Management of seizures

- Maintain airway as able—use a naso- or oropharyngeal airway if tolerated (an oropharyngeal airway may prove impossible to insert in a fitting athlete due to teeth clenching)
- Administer 15 L of oxygen as available
- Check for a pulse
- If fitting for more than 2 min
- Obtain IV access if possible and check using a blood glucose monitor (BM)
  - If IV access is obtained then administer 0.1 mg/kg lorazepam
  - If no IV access then use 0.5 mg/kg diazepam pr or 0.5 mg buccal midazolam and try again for IV access
- Phone an ambulance if fitting for more than 5 min
- If still fitting after 10 min
  - If IV access is obtained then administer 0.1mg/kg lorazepam
  - If still no IV access then use a further 0.5mg/kg diazepam PR or 0.5mg/kg buccal midazolam and try again for IV access
- ENSURE AMBULANCE HAS BEEN CALLED.
  (Adapted from APLS)

⚠ Limping child

The differential diagnosis for a child presenting with a limp is exceptionally varied and causes originating anywhere from the spine to the toe nails should be sought. Pain from the hip is often felt in the knee so hip pathology should always be considered in a child with knee pain.

Different causes will occur at different ages such as transient synovitis being more common in the under 10-year-olds and a slipped femoral epiphysis in the over 10-year-olds. The child may or may not complain of pain—indeed, the limp may be detected by the clinician or a concerned parent without the child even being aware of it. Fever is a most concerning symptom and septic arthritis should always be considered in such presentations.

Management will depend on the likely cause found via a thorough history and examination. In many cases, radiological and blood tests will not be required, and a wait and see plan may be put in place, as long as the child is reassessed regularly. In more complex cases or where there is any doubt as to the pathology then specialist referral for imaging and further investigation will be required.

Potential causes of a limping child

▶ In *all* age groups *always* consider the possibility of non-accidental injury (NAI).

- *Age 0–4:*
  - Trauma—toddlers fracture (#)
  - soft tissue injury (STI) to foot
  - Septic arthritis/Osteomyelitis
  - Transient synovitis
  - Hair tourniquet
  - Juvenile rheumatoid arthritis
  - Rarely—malignancy.
- *Age 4–10:*
  - Trauma—fracture or STI to lower limb including epiphyseal injuries
  - Septic arthritis/osteomyelitis
  - Transient synovitis
  - Perthes disease
  - Leukaemia
  - Juvenile rheumatoid arthritis.
- *Age 10–18:*
  - Trauma—fracture or STI to lower limb including epiphyseal injuries, and avulsion fractures
  - Slipped upper femoral capital epiphysis (SUFE)
  - Septic arthritis/osteomyelitis
  - Leukaemia and malignancies
  - Juvenile ankylosing spondylitis.

History

Important factors in the history include:

- Trauma: If so then what was the mechanism
- Associated fever: should raise concern over infective cause such as septic arthritis. Mandates referral for blood and imaging work-up
- Associated night pain
- Associated systemic upset or weight loss
- Multiple joints affected
- Previous history: perthes is bilateral in approximately 15%
- Family history of joint diseases/HLA B27.

►► Remember to be careful to allow the parent or child to answer without direct questioning initially. It is all too easy to be distracted by an 'injury' where the parents or child tries to help you by attributing the symptoms to a possible trauma when, in fact, this is a red herring.

►► Night pain and weight loss are vague symptoms, but should raise concerns of a potentially significant aetiology, such as malignancy.

Examination

The examination made will be directed depending on whether there has been a history of trauma or not.

- In any case of a traumatic injury the athlete should be assessed using the ABC approach and a focused assessment made thereafter of the injured limb including the joints above and below the injured area.
- In atraumatic limping, examination should include a general examination of the athlete to include pulse and temperature.
- The child's weight should also be taken.
- Assessment of the child's gait should be made followed by an examination, starting with the lumbar spine and working down to assess the pelvis, hips femur, knee, lower limb then the ankle, foot, and finally the toes if a cause for the limp has not been found by this point.
- Each joint should be assessed using the standard joint examination principles of look, feel, and move.
- Symmetry should be assessed by examining the unaffected leg as this will help to clarify the normal range of movement and also allow you to assess for polyarthropathy too.

Investigations

- Will depend on the clinical findings and the working diagnosis.
- In any child with a fever and a restricted range of hip movement, referral should be made for a work-up of laboratory tests to include full blood count (FBC), c-reactive protein (CRP), X-ray and possible ultrasound (US) with a view to hip joint aspiration depending on local policies.

Septic arthritis

⚠ Septic arthritis is an orthopaedic emergency.

- Suspect in any child with a fever and a painful/inability to weight bear (Note: there may be no fever)
- Usually *Staph. aureus*

- Can occur in any age, but the majority of patients are around 3 years old
- May be little in the way of clinical findings of erythema, warm joint, or swelling. Child may hold the hip flexed abducted and rotate externally
- Immediately refer for blood tests and imaging followed by antibiotics and joint washout.

Perthes' disease

- Aseptic (avascular) necrosis of the femoral head
- The classic cause of a 'painless' limp. Aetiology unknown
- Also known as (Legg–Calve–Perthes' disease)
- Boys are affected more than girls by a factor of about ×4
- Peak age is usually in the 4–10-year-old group
- Occurs bilaterally in about 10–15% so ask about previous history
- Pain may be referred to the anterior thigh or the knee
- Pain may be found maximally on internal rotation and abduction
- Diagnosis is confirmed with X-ray
- Treatment may either be conservative with splinting and traction or be surgical via an osteotomy. Either way the aim is to maximize the femoral head regaining its correct anatomical shape
- Long-term outcomes vary depending on the extent of necrosis and age the condition develops with best outcomes in the younger population
- Return to sport can be considered once the child is pain free and X-ray appearances confirm healing of the femoral head.

Slipped upper femoral capital epiphysis

- Boys affected more than girls by a factor of about ×3
- Increased incidence in obese children and some medical conditions, such as metabolic disorders of growth, hypogonadism, and hypothyroidism. Peak age is usually in the 10–17-year-old group
- May occur bilaterally in about 40% (usually within 2 years of the first hip) resulting in some athletes opting for prophylactic fixation of an unaffected hip
- Progressive pain in hip/groin. Pain on internal rotation and abduction
- Treatment is invariably surgical after X-ray diagnosis
- Crutches and graded weight-bearing for at least 2 months
- Return to play once pain free. Some advocate X-ray confirmation of the physis closing prior to return to contact sport.

Transient synovitis of the hip

- This is a particularly common cause of a limp in children (especially under the age of 10 years old)
- It is best considered a diagnosis of exclusion, i.e. there is absolutely nothing to suggest a septic arthritis as discussed before
- Aetiology is thought to be secondary to a viral infection and, as such, there may be a history of a recent or ongoing coryzal illness
- Investigations are non-specific with only mild if any elevation in inflammatory markers. X-ray will be normal and is not routinely required
- US will diagnose the effusion, but there is no distinction between the causes for the effusion, i.e. septic arthritis
- Management is symptomatic with rest simple analgesia and anti-inflammatories.

⊕: Head injury

Paediatric head injuries are common. Over 500,000 children present to EDs across the UK each year as a result of head injury. The majority of these will be 'minor' implying that there is no serious intracranial pathology.

⚠ However, 1:500 children initially classified as having a 'minor head injury' will actually ultimately have serious intracranial pathology.

Initial assessment of the head injured child

▶▶ The initial assessment of a child with a head injury is no different to that of an adult with a head injury (see 🕮 also p.116)

History is again key.

- What was the mechanism of injury?
- Was the child unconscious? If so for how long?
- Has the child vomited?
- Did they suffer a seizure (pre- or post-injury)?
- Have they been amnesic and is so, for how long?

These questions form the basic framework for the decision-making criteria about whether the child needs to go to hospital and needs imaging.

Examination is again primarily used to both assess and treat injuries as they are found.

- Protect the cervical spine and assess the airway
- Reassurance will be required so talk calmly to the child
- Involve the parents if present (*Do not*, however, allow them to move the child until you have completed your assessment.)
- Ensure assistance has been called for
- Proceed to assessing breathing and circulation (bear in mind the differences in normal values in differing age groups)
- Over the age of 5 years, the adult GCS assessment scoring system (see 🕮 p.116) or alternatively, the AVPU system can be used when assessing disability. Under the age of 5 an adjusted Glasgow Coma Score (GCS) system is used, although this is a rare sporting event and, as such, AVPU is recommended in this age group
- Log roll should be carried out as per the guidance detailed on 🕮 p.15:
  - If the child is small it may be more appropriate to use 2 persons to log roll the child rather than 3
  - This will depend on the length of the child and is really a judgment call
  - Best advice is that if the 3 persons standing to roll the child cannot place their hands appropriately because they are in each others way then only 2 will be required.

Head injury management

The way children with head injuries are managed has changed in recent years after the publication of guidelines such as NICE and SIGN 110, and CHALICE.

These papers have focused on the best methods of investigating these injuries—who to image and when. This guidance is invaluable to the pitchside clinician who can much more readily decide who to refer to hospital.

Indications for referral to the ED
- GCS <15 at initial assessment
- Post-traumatic seizure (generalized or focal)
- Focal neurological signs
- Signs of a skull fracture
- Loss of consciousness
- Sever and persistent headache
- Repeated vomiting (two or more occasions)
- Post-traumatic amnesia >5 min
- Retrograde amnesia >30 min
- High risk mechanism of injury
- Coagulopathy
- Clinical suspicion of NAI.

Indications for CT scan immediate
- GCS 13 or less in ED
- GCS 14 or 15/15, but witnessed the loss of consciousness (LOC) >5 min
- GCS 14 or 15/15, but suspicion of open or depressed skull #
- GCS 14 or 15/15, but focal neurology
- GCS 14 or 15/15, but basal skull #.

Indications to consider CT scan within 8 h
- GCS 14 or 15, but presence of bruise, swelling, or lac >5 cm
- GCS 14 or 15, and post-traumatic seizure (no history of epilepsy)
- GCS 14 or 15, and any amnesia lasting >5 min
- GCS 14 or 15, and a history of significant fall
- GCS 14 or 15, and 3 or more discrete episodes of vomiting
- GCS 14 or 15, and abnormal drowsiness (slow to respond).

Return to sport guidelines

The guidance detailed in 📖 p.124 is applicable to children aged 10 and above. Further research is being undertaken to provide evidence on the safest way to return a child to sport in the ages below this. At present the guidance as laid out in 📖 p.124, i.e. rest followed by a graded return to full activities is the suggested advice.

Useful drug doses in children

See Table 18.2.

Table 18.2 Useful drugs dosages to consider

Paracetamol po	loading dose 20 mg/kg then 10–15 mg/kg
Ibuprofen po	loading dose of 10 mg/kg then 7 mg/kg
Lorazepam IV	0.1 mg/kg
Diazepam pr	0.5 mg/kg
Morphine IV	0.1 mg/kg
Adrenaline in cardiac arrest	0.1 mL/kg of 1:10,000

Further reading

British Thoracic Guidelines/Scottish Intercollegiate Guidelines Network (2008, revised 2011). Available at: ℘ www.sign.ac.uk/pdf/qrg101.pdf.

Wyatt JP, Illingworth RN, Graham CA, et al. (2006). *Oxford Handbook of Emergency Medicine*. Oxford: Oxford University Press.

Athletes with a disability

Introduction

Disability sport is the term used for any sport undertaken by someone with a disability (Table 19.1). It therefore covers a wide range of sports and athletes with 20 summer and 5 winter sports at Paralympic games.

Table 19.1 Sports undertaken by people with disabilities

Summer Paralympic sports				Winter sports
Archery	Football 5-a-side	Rowing	Volleyball (sitting)	Alpine skiing
Athletics	Football 7-a-side	Sailing	Wheelchair basketball	Biathlon
Boccia	Goalball	Shooting	Wheelchair fencing	Cross-country skiing
Cycling	Judo	Swimming	Wheelchair rugby	Ice sledge hockey
Equestrian	Powerlifting	Table tennis	Wheelchair tennis	Wheelchair curling

Five major impairment groups are recognized for the elite athletes in the Paralympics.
• Visual impairment
• Spinal-cord-related disability (congenital or acquired)
• Limb deficiencies (congenital or acquired)
• Cerebral palsy
• Les Autres (for athletes who do not fit into other categories).

Athletes with intellectual impairment will be reintroduced at the 2012 Paralympics in a limited number of sports following issues relating to classification systems, but are involved in a number of sports at the community level.

Athletes with disabilities can compete in a wide range of sports as part of the Paralympics, and a wider range of sports and activities within communities.

Principles of treatment

The principles of treatment for injuries are identical to those in able-bodied athletes. See 🕮 Chapter 2 for all injuries that follow the ABCDE approach.

Special considerations

- Knowledge of the regulations covering the sport is important, although outside the scope of this book (see www.paralympic.org for further information)
- Each individual sport will potentially use specialist equipment and a working knowledge of this equipment will be vital. For example, when working with athletes using wheelchairs, it is vital to know how to release the athletes quickly from their chairs in event of significant trauma
- Field of play recovery also needs consideration for each sport and should be practiced by the team prior to the commencement of events—e.g. in wheelchair events a crash involving a number of wheelchair athletes on a track will pose a significant challenge to most field-of-play medical response teams unless adequately rehearsed
- The nature of the injuries likely to be experienced depend on the nature of the sport—e.g. alpine skiing or sledge hockey with high impact collisions as compared with archery. However, it is important to note that a high index of suspicion is required, for fractures with minimal trauma in athletes with paralysis and consequent osteoporosis/osteopenia. For example, a sideways fall onto the lateral hip in a chair can result in hip fractures, although the forces involved do not appear significant
- Knowing the athletes you are caring for is always important, but not always possible. So understanding the different impairment groups involved in each sport will give an indication of the type of medical issues likely to be faced. However, in the Les Autres groups this can be challenging and, in athletes with rare conditions, the use of a textbook is important!
- Sometimes a condition will not only have physical limitations, but may have intellectual and emotional components, which need to be considered in the treatment of the athlete
- In athletes with intellectual impairment, consent to treatment can be an issue, which should be considered prior to participation
- There is often a higher incidence of epilepsy in these athletes and provision for this should be considered in the planning of an event
- The co-existence of other diseases and use of medications is more frequent in this group of athletes and these may affect response to injury. For example, tetraplegic athletes with limited respiratory reserve will deteriorate quicker with chest trauma than an able bodied athlete
- Skin care of the stump in amputee athletes needs careful consideration and repeated observation, to ensure that breakdown of the tissue does not occur
- There is also the potential for penetrating injuries if prosthesis breaks suddenly during an event.

:⚙: Autonomic dysreflexia

- This occurs in patients with a chronic or acute spinal cord lesion above T5–6
- It is an exaggerated increase in blood pressure (BP) as a result of a noxious stimulus below the level of the lesion
- The autonomic nervous system depends on a balance between the parasympthatic and sympathetic nervous systems
- The sympathetic system is associated with the fight or flight response, which includes:
  - Dilation of the pupil
  - Increase in heart rate
  - Vasoconstriction
  - Release of catecholamine hormones (adrenalin)
- The parasympathetic system produces opposite responses, which includes:
  - Constriction of the pupil
  - Decrease in heart rate
- The sympathetic and parasympathetic nerves have different pathways in the body with the sympathetic system having a major output between the 5th thoracic and 2nd lumbar segments of the spinal cord
- In a patient with a spinal cord lesion above the level of the 5th and 6th thoracic vertebrae, a painful stimulus below the level of the lesion will produce a response by the sympathetic system, which may result in:
  - Vasoconstriction
  - High BP
  - Pounding headache
  - Anxiety
  - Pallor
  - Goosebumps
- The skin changes will occur below the level of the lesion only
- The parasympathetic system is unable to counteract these effects below the level of the lesion and so produces bradycardia and flushing of the neck and face by vasodilation.

Symptoms of autonomic dysreflexia
- Anxiety
- Pounding headache
- Sweating
- Chest pain.

Signs of autonomic dysreflexia
- Flushing of face and neck
- Hypertension with bradycardia
- Possible cardiac arrythmias
- Dilated pupils
- Goosebumps below the level of the lesion
- Cold peripheries.

The baseline BP in a spinal cord patient is often relatively low and so a significant rise may not be appreciated—it is important to know the baseline BPs for all athletes at risk of this complication.

The increase in BP is a medical emergency, and prompt recognition and treatment is essential.

Causes

Any noxious stimuli below the level of the lesion can cause the condition. These may be painful, uncomfortable, or physically irritating. The most common cause is overfilling of the bladder followed by gas- or stool-filled bowel.

Causes in the bladder
- Retention
- Infection
- Over-filled collection system
- Calculi.

Causes in the bowel
- Constipation
- Digital stimulation
- Haemorrhoids and fissures
- Infection.

Causes in the skin
- Pressure sores
- In-growing toenail
- Burns
- Restrictive clothing below the level of the lesion
- Wrinkled clothing or pressure from a foreign body.

Other causes
Include:
- Sexual activity
- Menstrual cramps
- Injuries such as fractures.

Treatment

The most important treatment is the identification and removal of the stimulus. Sometimes this will be obvious, but it is recommended to ensure a thorough examination for the cause using a step approach. Always complete all steps.

Therefore:
- *Step 1:* check bladder
- *Step 2:* check bowel
- *Step 3:* check skin
- *Step 4:* check other.

Treatment is required to lower BP. This can be achieved with either:
• Nifedepine 10 mg (capsules that can be chewed or split into the mouth)
• Glyceryl trinitrate (GTN) spray.

During the initial management, arrangements should be made for transfer to hospital unless rapid resolution of the symptoms and signs are achieved.

Aggressive patients

Introduction

Aggressive or violent acts are often associated with sport. When people are brought together in competition, they demonstrate their physical and tactical supremacy within pre-established rules or laws of the game, but a strong desire to win may lead them to overlook these rules. This can lead to actions that endanger their opponents' well-being.

In professional sport, these acts tend to be highlighted by the media and sometimes appear to provoke violent acts by supporters who may be incensed or inappropriately inspired by the on-pitch activities.

Within a sporting environment, aggressive behaviour might not just be between competitors, but athletes might be aggressive to staff (including doctors) or even spectators

Effective communication with aggressive or violent patients, whether in a sporting environment or not, is obviously challenging. It is essential to bear in mind one's own safety and to proceed cautiously when engaging such patients.

Explaining aggression and violence

Aggression and violence in a sporting environment has a number of possible causes or precipitating factors (see Box 20.1 for relevant definitions).

- *Misunderstanding or misinterpretation:*
  - Lack of language skills
  - Cultural differences
  - Misinterpretation of body language
- *Personality types involved:*
  - Competitive, fearless
  - Accustomed to violence (on the field of play), but unable to make a distinction when they cross over the boundary where such behaviour is unacceptable
- *Emotions:*
  - Disappointment
  - Frustration
  - Anger—loss, failure, blaming others
- *Confusion:* consider medical causes especially hypoglycaemia:
  - Pain (e.g. From sports injuries)
  - Brain injury
  - Metabolic (e.g. dehydration, heat exhaustion)
  - Infective
  - Neoplastic causes (e.g. brain tumour)
  - Drugs—stimulants, alcohol, or anabolic steroids
- *Mental illness:*
  - Psychosis (e.g. due to schizophrenia or bipolar illness)
  - Depression
  - Anxiety state or panic attack.

Box 20.1 Definitions

- *Aggression:* behaviour in which there is intent to harm or cause damage, though this may not be a conscious decision
- *Violence:* physically harmful or damaging behaviour, where there is pre-meditation or planning
- *Assertive:* behaviour associated with trying to control a situation, but with no intent to cause harm or damage

Preventing aggression or violence in athletes

It is often possible to prevent potential acts of aggression or violence from escalating. Engendering mutual trust and respect is important to building a good doctor–patient relationship. It is advisable to:

- Consult out of the media spotlight and 'public eye' as much as possible
- Consult in a room suitable for medical purposes where possible
- Explore the needs and expectations of the athlete sensitively
- Explain the reasons for carrying out any action or procedure and ensure agreement or consent so that actions may not be misconstrued (e.g. as an assault.)
- Remain impartial—do not appear to take sides with management, coach, other players, or the opposition
- Arrange a chaperone.

Facilities

- Sports physicians should impress upon management that it is essential to provide a suitable medical room, the layout of which should be planned bearing in mind dealing with aggressive or violent patients
- An easy route of escape for the doctor and a panic alarm facility should be available with other staff aware of the expectations if the alarm is sounded.

Early warning signs

Changes in character or behaviour

- The player's on- or off-pitch behaviour may change before their actions turn aggressive. These changes may be subtle or obvious
- Typically, dehydrated or heat-affected players lose position or role sense in their team, and the sports physician should assess and manage their condition appropriately
- There may be a character change in a sportsman suffering the delayed effects of a head injury
- Appropriate, urgent assessment, investigation, and management can prevent an even more catastrophic outcome.

Education

- The governing bodies of sports have a duty to educate players about the dangers of aggressive behaviour in their sport and to encourage the ethics of fair play
- The doctors involved in sports must play their part by upholding the laws of the sport and spirit of the game. They must also adhere rigidly to the professional ethics and regulations that govern their medical profession.

Dealing with aggressive or violent athletes

Situations can arise rapidly and unexpectedly in which a doctor will feel threatened by an athlete. It is important that the doctor's own behaviour remain non-aggressive and does not lead to the situation escalating with significant injury to doctor, athlete, anyone else, or damage to property.

The following tips may be helpful:

- Use calm tones
- Use reassuring words
- Body language:
  - The doctor should let his arms hanging down
  - Have the palms turned into an open position
- Move towards an exit and away from aggressor
- Express empathy—e.g. 'I'm sorry you feel like this' or 'I want to understand why you feel like that.'
- Express willingness to help—'Tell me how I can make the situation better.'
- Avoid pointing, confrontation, staring, arguing, or raising one's voice.

Help and restraint

- The doctor must use their discretion as to when to summon help with a panic alarm, phone, or by shouting
- Having sufficient other bodies available will be essential to bring the situation under control if the athlete is intent on violent acts
- Those trained in restraint and crowd control (e.g. the police) would be valuable, although the familiar faces of other squad members or support staff might be more calming to the athlete.

Record keeping

When the doctor has achieved control of the situation, they should make comprehensive notes and involve appropriate other parties, such as:

- Psychiatrist
- Police
- Sports club or governing body officials
- Athlete's family.

There may be situations whereby the confidentiality of the doctor–patient relationship has to be breached. Each case will be unique and the merits and drawbacks of breaking confidentiality must be considered. If there is ethical uncertainty, it is advisable to obtain professional advice (e.g. from one's professional registration body) before deciding how best to proceed.

Summary

- Aggressive and violent behaviour may be present in a sports environment
- Some aggressive acts result from circumstance due to the sport, but others may originate in a mental or physical illness of the athlete
- Sports doctor must prepare themselves to deal with situations where their own well-being is threatened by an aggressive athlete
- Sports doctors must be vigilant for early signs in athletes that might lead to aggressive or violent behaviour.

Breaking bad news

Introduction

A sports doctor will occasionally be responsible for imparting bad news to an athlete or participant within the sporting arena.

This information can have a significant impact on a patient's fitness to play, general health, or career earnings.

Selected examples include:

- Informing an athlete that they cannot compete in a major competition due to injury
- That their injury is so severe that it may threaten their future involvement in competitive sport.

Although the environment a sports doctor works in may be different from that of a hospital, hospice, or community clinic, the principles of 'breaking bad news' remain the same. The importance of doing this fundamental task well cannot be overstated.

General principles

Prepare ('before')

- Bad news should ideally be communicated in person. Traditionally, this is done by a senior and experienced medical doctor, but that may not always be possible
- It is never a pleasant task, but do not avoid meeting the patient or leave them 'stranded' without any news. Anticipation can be worse than the actual news itself!
- If it is your responsibility to tell the patient and they are not immediately present, ask a receptionist or colleague to contact the patient and make an appointment to see you. (Asking a third person to arrange this appointment ensures that the news does not get 'leaked' if the patient quizzes you, and gives you the opportunity to create an ideal environment beforehand in which to convey the news.)
- Alternatively, it may sometimes be appropriate to call the patient yourself if they already have an inkling of what the problem is and are expecting a telephone call from you
- Follow this up by arranging a subsequent face-to-face discussion to talk about their problems in greater detail
- The patient may like to be accompanied by their coach or family member. Allow them to do so
- If dealing with a child or teenager, it is ideal if you can have the parent/s present when you convey the information. This may not always be possible, e.g. when a child or teenager has travelled to a training camp or competition in a foreign country
- Remember that if you are asked to discuss the medical condition with a concerned third party, e.g. relatives or carers other than the parent or guardian of a child, you must have the patient's consent if he/she is in a position to give it
- Familiarize yourself with the facts as far as possible. If discussing imaging results, consider discussing the imaging investigations in detail with a radiologist beforehand. It can also be valuable to have the images available to show the athlete
- Try to anticipate the types of questions you may be asked and consider how you might answer them. Have a clear plan for dealing with the problem—this may involve a specialist opinion, detailed rehabilitation plans or structured advice for the future
- Ensure a private, quiet environment where possible
- Create 'protected time'
- Turn off your mobile phone or pager
- Do not appear to be in a hurry
- Allow time for the patient and others present to ask questions.

Communicate ('during')

- Establish previous knowledge
  - What does the patient know already?
  - What were they expecting?
- A 'warning shot across the bow' to prepare them may be helpful. This can include phrases such as 'I'm sorry to say it is rather bad news'. Allow a moment for this to sink in
- Establish how much detail the patient wants to know
- Be aware of subtle visual and verbal cues. This is helpful in establishing a rapport and trust if this is the first time the sports doctor is meeting the patient
- Use language that the patient will understand. The level of comprehension will depend upon the age and educational background of the patient, but in general, avoid jargon, technical terms, and abbreviations
- If appropriate, structure the discussion into stages, such as diagnosis, implications, management (and prognosis in the case of patients with a terminal illness. This situation will be rare within a sporting context)
- Be aware that patients often take in only a fraction of the information conveyed to them initially and repetition may be necessary
- It is not essential to cover all aspects in great detail immediately
- Attempt to convey optimism, but still be honest and realistic, especially when dealing with a patient's expectations
- Expect the unexpected:
  - Patients can react in all sorts of ways to receiving bad news
  - Be empathic and do not be judgmental
- Observe to see how the patient is coping, but resist the urge to 'make everything better immediately'. Patients need time to let the news sink in
- Listen to your patient for their thoughts, ideas, and any immediate questions they may have
- Do not expect to deal with everything in one session
- Know when to conclude the consultation. 'Would you like to leave it for now and we can discuss it again when you are feeling ready?' Bear in mind they may wish you to speak to someone else or have someone with them for the next meeting
- Agree the short-term plan and further follow-up.

Conclude ('after')

- Finish with a brief summary and try to conclude on an optimistic note where possible. No matter how bad the news is, it is important that you do not rob the patient of all hope!
- Give appropriate written material or patient information leaflets if you have some available
- Inter-professional communication may be very helpful to ensure the patient is well supported. In the sporting arena, this will usually include coaches, managers, and relevant team staff:
  - Inform other colleagues involved in the patient's care if appropriate, but ensure the athlete's consent is obtained beforehand

- • The input of a sports psychologist can be very helpful for aiding the elite athlete in coping with disappointment, injury, and the often arduous process of rehabilitation
- Respect the patient's right to confidentiality at all times
- Some athletes will cope with bad news by 'externalizing' blame—for example, blaming a physiotherapist or other doctor for a delay in diagnosis or what they perceive to be substandard care. Be careful not to 'add fuel to the fire' with careless remarks!
- Record clear and contemporaneous notes of the discussion. You or your colleagues may need to refer to it in future
- Imparting bad news can be an emotional (and often difficult) experience for the doctor, as well as the patient, so take a moment to recognize this and collect your thoughts before moving on to the next task.

Further reading

Knott, L. (2008). *Breaking Bad News.* ℘ www.patient.co.uk.

Midgley, S.J., Heather, N., Davis, J.B. (2001). Levels of aggression among a group of anabolic-androgenic steroid users. *Med Sci Law* **41**(4): 309–14.

Pope, H.G.J., Katz, D.L. (1990). Homicide and near-homicide by anabolic steroid users. *J Clin Psychiat* **51**(1): 28–31.

Simpson, C. (2004). When hope makes us vulnerable: a discussion of patient-healthcare provider in-teractions in the context of hope. *Bioethics* **18**(5): 428–47.

Tenenbaum, G.E., Singer R.N, Duda J. (1997). Aggression and violence in sport: an ISSP position stand. *J Sports Med Phys Fitness* **37**(2): 146–50.

VandeKieft, G.K. (2001). Breaking bad news. *Am Fam Physician* **64**(12): 1975–8.

Websites

(2009). Useful resources for UK Health Professionals. *Breaking Bad News.* ℘ www.breakingbadnews.co.uk website. 2009.

Communication

Introduction

Excellent communication skills and the ability to work alongside colleagues are essential qualities for all clinical doctors, particularly those working within the sporting team. Both these skills are specifically mentioned in the General Medical Council (GMC) guidance for doctors *Good Medical Practice*.

The nature of the multidisciplinary team in performance sport necessitates clear strategic direction and definition of individual's roles. Within the sporting environment, the medical team is one part of the overall performance team.

The performance team is the ultimate multidisciplinary team and is often composed of individuals with very different professional, educational, social, and sporting backgrounds. The knowledge and skills of these individuals, all of which are critical to team or athlete success, are not always aligned in fundamental approach. There is also the potential for significant overlap of roles and responsibilities.

Composition of multidisciplinary team in sporting environment

- Athlete
- Coach, manager, selectors
- Strength and conditioning coach
- Administrators
- Sport and exercise medicine physician
- *Therapists:* physiotherapist, chiropractors, osteopaths, soft tissue therapists, others
- Nutritionist
- Physiologist
- Psychologist
- Biomechanist
- Podiatrist
- *External consultants:* radiologists, orthopaedic surgeons, others.

Challenges to effective communication in this environment

- Athlete medical confidentiality
- Lack of defined roles and responsibilities
- Essential requirement for strong relationships of trust between team members
- Ability to travel abroad and spend prolonged periods of time with other team members
- Different medical opinions given to athlete/coach from members within the multidisciplinary team
- Different medical information given to athlete/coach from external medical opinions (solicited or unsolicited)
- Time pressures
- Media requests
- Electronic notes databases.

Communication: athlete confidentiality

As stated in *Good Medical Practice*, patients have 'a right to expect that information about them will be held in confidence by their doctors'. This is fundamental to all medical practice and is essential to maintain the professional integrity and trust of all athletes in the physician's care.

However, disclosure of medical information to non-medical personnel in the multi-disciplinary team is necessary for the performance team to function effectively. There are some practical suggestions for dealing with this issue in the sporting context.

Athlete contracts and consent

- These should state that medical information that impacts on the athlete's ability to perform will be disclosed to the head coach/manager
- The physician should still request consent after each consultation before disclosing medical information to coaches
- Athletes may withdraw consent at any time and for any particular condition. In this case, the doctor should inform the head coach that consent for disclosure has been withdrawn.

Transfer of information

- The relevant medical information should be passed in a secure format to only the individuals that need to know for purposes of team selection or rehabilitation planning
- These individuals should be made aware that information is not to be passed on without further athlete consent and must be stored securely
- Any transfer of information to the media should be done with athlete consent.

Meetings

- Attendance of both the coach and athlete at clinical reviews or at team meetings can be a useful way of involving coaches in receiving medical information
- Regular team meetings between the head coach and lead medical officer are invaluable.

Other athletes

- The medical team must have a private room facility for reviewing patients if desired
- Members of the medical team should never discuss an athlete's medical issues with other athletes or in the patient's absence in communal training or rehabilitation areas
- Professionalism should be maintained at all times.

Communication: defining roles

Multidisciplinary teams in elite sport are usually composed of individuals with enthusiasm and intelligence, diverse skill sets, a passion for the sport and a willingness to perform duties not specifically recognized as part of their job description.

Indeed, this is usually encouraged as part of being an excellent team member. Such energy, passion, and intelligence can, however, lead to individuals offering advice and information regarding another team member's area of expertise.

Although useful and appropriate if channelled skillfully, there are a number of possible −ive consequences. First, the athlete can receive mixed messages, which can be both detrimental to their understanding or their rehabilitation goals. This type of communication can also undermine practitioners in their area of expertise and lead to sub-standard overall care.

Recommendations for good practice can include:

- *Clearly define roles and responsibilities of team members:*
  - With regards to athletes' sustaining a new injury, the role and responsibility of the team doctor might be defined primarily as diagnosis, investigation, and early intervention, or management
  - The physiotherapist's primary role and responsibility may be defined as the rehabilitation or exercise prescription through to return to sport
  - As the team relationships and dynamics evolve and become more sophisticated, both the doctor and the physiotherapist will communicate appropriately with each other to influence each practitioner's primary responsibility
- *Encourage and facilitate discussion within the multidisciplinary team:*
  - Facilitate and support communication within the team with both formal meetings and informal conversations
  - Do not comment directly to athletes regarding issues that come under other team members (coaches or medical practitioners) areas of expertise
  - Individual disagreements should be discussed by the practitioners concerned and within the team, never with the athlete directly.

Communication: external opinions

Effective referral to external consultants is an essential requirement for a medical physician to be successful in an elite sporting environment. It is important to establish excellent communication and relationships.

Two examples are provided; although it is recognized that expertise from other specialties may also be warranted.

Radiologists

- It is useful for the athlete's physician to have an excellent relationship with a small number of local radiologists
- The sports physician should be aware of the individual nuances in reporting
- The sports physician's expectation of the nature of communication from the radiologist should be clearly defined
- To ensure good record keeping, written reports should always be produced and filed in the patient's notes, even if a verbal report has been discussed beforehand with the athlete or athlete's physician
- It is usually inappropriate for the radiologist to communicate with the athlete regarding diagnosis, rehabilitation plans, or healing time frames.

Surgeons

The choice of surgical referral should be made by the athlete's sports physician after discussion with the athlete.

The decision to refer should be based on a number of considerations including:

- Detailed awareness of the procedures the surgeon can offer
- Expertise of the surgeon
- The surgeon's understanding of elite sport and experience with elite athletes
- Accessibility
- The surgeon's ability to communicate appropriately with the athlete and coach, and to involve the managing medical team in decision-making
- It is usually helpful to discuss the referral verbally with the surgeon prior to the consultation. This should be followed with a professional written correspondence. It is ideal that the managing sports physician attends the surgical consultation.

Communication when travelling abroad or to major championships

Major championships and travelling abroad provide many additional pressures that require effective communication within the multidisciplinary team.

- Provision should be made for appropriate written documentation regarding athlete's medical presentations. A database with an on- and offline facility is particularly useful to maintain athlete's medical notes
- Daily clinical meetings are particularly to be recommended:
  - The timing of these will depend on the competition schedule and the timing of the team management meeting
  - If possible, the clinical meeting should directly precede the team management meeting so that the medical representative is fully updated for the team management meeting
- Individual practitioners should communicate their own needs to the leader of the medical team
- Travelling abroad with a team can be an exhausting activity and individuals should be mindful of keeping their productivity and effectiveness high by taking appropriate nutrition, rest, and recovery.

Communication with the media: press releases

Sports physicians working as elite team doctors or governing body medical officers will often come under pressure to divulge medical information about their patients to the media.

An awareness of the requirement for confidentiality and professional obligation to respect it is essential at all times.

If you are asked to provide information about patients, you must:

- Inform patients about the disclosure, or check that they have already received information about it
- Anonymize data where unidentifiable data will serve the purpose
- Be satisfied that patients know about disclosures necessary to provide their care, or for local clinical audit of that care, that they can object to these disclosures, but have not done so
- Seek patients' express consent to disclosure of information, where identifiable data is needed for any purpose other than the provision of care or for clinical audit—save in the exceptional circumstances
- Keep disclosures to the minimum necessary
- Keep up to date with and observe the requirements of statute and common law, including data protection legislation.

Sporting organizations vary in their approach to informing the public of the injuries and illnesses that afflict their players. Most appoint media relations officers who will often communicate messages to interested journalists by e-mail.

- The media officer will be tasked to gauge the public perceptions of the organization by reading the newspapers, and listening to interviews and comment on radio and television
- They will also be best placed to advise the medical officer about possible misconceptions.

Doctors may have the opportunity to influence the content of such press releases.

- A proactive approach is recommended for the club doctor who should check the content is accurate and that the wording has the full consent of the player before submitting it
- The doctor should try to anticipate what will happen as a consequence of releasing this information and the press release should be written in a language that is readily understood by the non-medical public
- There is no benefit to the doctor being quoted in the press release
- It is generally better that the statement comes from the organization, club, or governing body.

Consider that club officials (e.g. coach, captain, performance manager, chief executive) and other parties with vested interests (e.g. agents, sponsors) may need to be briefed (with the patient's full consent) before the statement goes public.

The press release should be as complete as possible, because any omissions will attract further questions from curious and usually persistent journalists.

When preparing a press release, consider providing the following information:

- What happened? (circumstances, problem, diagnosis)
- What is happening? (current management)
- What is going to happen? (future management plan)
- How bad is it? (severity/prognosis, i.e. predict missed matches, key events).

Media interviews

Occasionally, the media may want to interview the medical professional looking after an elite sports-person who has become injured or unwell. Should an interview be agreed, the doctor should prepare carefully.

When preparing for interviews with media:
- Request recorded live interviews
- Rehearse and know your intended message well
- Agree with the athlete the information they consent for you to impart in the interview
- Prepare a response to questions that are not anticipated or covered by the athlete's consent, e.g. 'I am not in a position to be able to comment on that at this time'
- Ask the interviewer to brief you on intended questions in advance
- Rehearse with the interviewer, if possible
- Tidy up your appearance
- Consider the proposed interview environment—minimize loud background sounds and sights that may give an unprofessional image.

In the interview (or press conference):
- Look and sound confident
- Repeat your prepared message
- Anticipate potential pitfalls
- Do not breach confidentiality providing information beyond that which is covered by the athlete's consent
- Avoid commenting on unprepared issues. You may need to state and restate, 'I am not in a position to be able to comment on that at this time'.

Further reading

Gregory, P.L., Seah, R., Pollock, N. (2008). What to tell the media—or not: consensus guide-lines for sports physicians. *Br J Sports Med* **42**(10): 485–8.

General Medical Council. (2006). *Good Medical Practice*. London: GMC.

BOA statement. (2000). The British Olympic Association's position statement on athlete confidentiality. *Br J Sports Med* **34**: 71–2.

Index